CONTENTS

Chapter 1: Introduction to Senior Wellness — 1

Chapter 2: Understanding Aging and the Body — 4

Chapter 3: Nutrition Essentials for Seniors — 8

Chapter 4: Staying Active at Every Age — 12

Chapter 5: Mental Health and Cognitive Well-being — 17

Chapter 6: Managing Chronic Conditions — 22

Chapter 7: Social Connections and Community Engagement — 28

Chapter 8: Preventive Healthcare Measures — 34

Chapter 9: Holistic Approaches to Aging — 41

Chapter 10: Adapting to Change and Embracing Resilience — 47

Chapter 11: Fostering Mental and Emotional Well-being — 53

Chapter 12: Embracing a Vibrant and Active Lifestyle — 60

Chapter 13: Practical Tips for Everyday Living — 66

Chapter 14: Navigating Healthcare Decisions and Advocacy — 72

Chapter 15: Cultivating Social Connections and Community Engagement — 78

Chapter 16: Nourishing Body and Mind: Holistic Approaches to Senior Nutrition — 84

Chapter 17: Embracing Fulfillment and Joy in Your Senior Years — 90

Chapter 18: Embracing the Fullness of Senior Life - A Recap — 95

CHAPTER 1: INTRODUCTION TO SENIOR WELLNESS

Embracing a Healthy and Fulfilling Senior Lifestyle

As the years advance, the pursuit of health and wellness takes center stage in our lives. Aging is a natural part of the human experience, and with it comes a unique set of challenges and opportunities. This chapter serves as a foundational guide, laying the groundwork for the importance of senior wellness and exploring the key elements that contribute to a fulfilling and healthy lifestyle in your later years.

The Significance of Senior Wellness

Embracing a Positive Perspective

Aging is often accompanied by societal stereotypes and misconceptions that can impact how individuals approach their senior years. It's crucial to break free from negative stereotypes and embrace a positive perspective on aging. The senior years can be a time of wisdom, growth, and new experiences. By prioritizing wellness, you can ensure that these years are not just lived but lived well.

Understanding the Holistic Approach

Senior wellness goes beyond mere physical health. It encompasses mental, emotional, and social well-being. A holistic approach to wellness acknowledges the interconnectedness of these aspects, recognizing that each plays a vital role in achieving a high quality of life. By addressing these dimensions collectively, individuals can enhance their overall well-being and truly thrive in their senior years.

The Aging Process and the Body

Physiological Changes

As we age, the body undergoes various physiological changes. Understanding these changes is crucial for proactively managing health. From a gradual decline in muscle mass to changes in bone density and a slowing metabolism, these transformations require attention and adaptation. However, with the right knowledge and lifestyle adjustments, seniors can navigate these changes with grace and maintain a vibrant and active lifestyle.

Importance of Regular Health Check-ups

Regular health check-ups become increasingly important in the senior years. These appointments provide an opportunity for early detection and prevention of potential health issues. From blood pressure monitoring to cholesterol checks and cancer screenings, staying proactive in healthcare significantly contributes to maintaining optimal well-being.

Setting the Stage for a Wellness Journey

Personal Reflection on Wellness Goals

Before delving into specific wellness strategies, it's essential for seniors to reflect on their personal goals and aspirations. What does a healthy and fulfilling life look like for you? Whether it's staying active to enjoy outdoor activities or maintaining strong social connections, understanding your unique priorities sets the foundation for a tailored wellness plan.

Building a Supportive Network

Embarking on a wellness journey is often more successful with a support network in place. This network may include healthcare professionals, family members, friends, and community resources. Cultivating a supportive environment ensures that individuals have the guidance and encouragement needed to navigate the challenges and celebrate the successes of their wellness journey.

Conclusion

This introductory chapter lays the groundwork for an enriching exploration of senior wellness. By embracing a positive perspective, understanding the aging process, and setting personal wellness goals, seniors can embark on a journey that prioritizes health and vitality. The subsequent chapters will delve into specific aspects of senior wellness, providing practical guidance and actionable steps to foster a life of fulfillment and well-being.

In the chapters to come, we will explore nutrition essentials, exercise routines, mental health strategies, and much more. The journey to vitality beyond years begins here, and with the right knowledge and mindset, seniors can navigate their wellness path with confidence and enthusiasm

CHAPTER 2: UNDERSTANDING AGING AND THE BODY

Embracing Change and Nurturing Wellness Through the Years

As we gracefully transition through the years, our bodies undergo a natural and intricate aging process. This chapter aims to shed light on the physiological changes that accompany aging, empowering seniors with knowledge to navigate these transformations. Understanding the nuances of aging is fundamental to cultivating a lifestyle that supports overall health and well-being.

The Physiology of Aging

Muscle Mass and Strength:

As we age, there is a gradual decline in muscle mass and strength. This can lead to challenges in maintaining balance and stability. However, incorporating strength training exercises into your routine can mitigate this decline, helping to preserve muscle mass and support overall mobility.

Bone Density:

Bone density tends to decrease with age, making bones more susceptible to fractures. Adequate calcium intake, along with weight-bearing exercises like walking or dancing, plays a crucial role in maintaining bone health. Regular bone density screenings can also provide insights into potential concerns.

Metabolism:

Metabolism tends to slow down as we age, affecting the body's ability to burn calories efficiently. This shift can contribute to weight gain. To counteract this, adopting a balanced diet and staying physically active become essential components of maintaining a healthy weight.

Hormonal Changes:

Hormonal changes, especially in women during menopause, can impact various aspects of health. Understanding and managing these changes, perhaps with the guidance of healthcare professionals, can help mitigate associated symptoms and support overall well-being.

The Role of Chronic Inflammation

Chronic inflammation is a common factor in many age-related diseases. It's the body's response to stress, injury, or prolonged exposure to harmful substances. While acute inflammation is a natural and protective response, chronic inflammation can contribute to conditions such as heart disease, diabetes, and arthritis.

Anti-Inflammatory Diet:

Adopting an anti-inflammatory diet rich in fruits, vegetables, whole grains, and omega-3 fatty acids can help manage inflammation. Foods like berries, leafy greens, and fatty fish have anti-inflammatory properties that support overall health.

Regular Exercise:

Physical activity is a powerful tool in controlling inflammation. Engaging in regular exercise not only helps maintain a healthy weight but also reduces inflammation and promotes cardiovascular health. Low-impact activities like swimming or cycling can be particularly beneficial for seniors.

The Importance of Flexibility and Mobility

Joint Health:

Maintaining joint health is crucial for overall mobility. Incorporating stretching exercises and activities like yoga can enhance flexibility and reduce the risk of joint-related issues. It's essential to listen to your body and adapt exercises to your individual needs and capabilities.

Posture and Balance:

With aging, there is an increased risk of changes in posture and balance. This can lead to a higher likelihood of falls. Practicing exercises that focus on balance, such as tai chi or specific balance drills, can help mitigate these risks and enhance overall stability.

Adapting Lifestyle Choices for Healthy Aging

Hydration:

As we age, the sensation of thirst may decrease, leading to dehydration. Staying adequately hydrated is vital for maintaining cognitive function, supporting digestion, and regulating body temperature. Seniors should be mindful of their water intake and incorporate hydrating foods like fruits and vegetables into their diet.

Smoking Cessation:

If applicable, quitting smoking is one of the most impactful steps towards better health. Smoking contributes to various health issues, including respiratory problems and heart disease. Seeking support through smoking cessation programs can significantly improve overall well-being.

Navigating Cognitive Changes

Brain Health:

Cognitive changes are a natural part of aging, but proactive steps can be taken to support brain health. Engaging in mentally stimulating activities, such as puzzles, reading, or learning new skills, helps maintain cognitive function. Additionally, staying socially active and connected has been linked to a lower risk of cognitive decline.

Memory Techniques:

Implementing memory techniques, such as creating associations or utilizing mnemonic devices, can be helpful in managing age-related memory changes. Regular mental exercises, combined with a healthy lifestyle, contribute to maintaining cognitive sharpness.

Seeking Professional Guidance

Importance of Regular Check-ups:

Regular health check-ups are crucial for monitoring and addressing potential health issues. Senior citizens should work closely with healthcare professionals to create a personalized healthcare plan, taking into account individual health history and potential risk factors.

Consulting Specialists:

Specialists such as geriatricians, nutritionists, and physical therapists can provide targeted guidance. Consulting with these professionals ensures that seniors receive specialized care and advice tailored to their unique needs and challenges.

Conclusion

Understanding the aging process empowers seniors to take proactive steps in nurturing their well-being. Embracing change, adopting healthy lifestyle choices, and seeking professional guidance form the cornerstone of a fulfilling and vibrant senior life. In the chapters that follow, we will delve into specific aspects of senior wellness, providing practical tips and actionable strategies to navigate the aging journey with grace and vitality. Remember, aging is not a hindrance but a new chapter filled with opportunities for growth, learning, and optimal well-being.

CHAPTER 3: NUTRITION ESSENTIALS FOR SENIORS

Nourishing Your Body, Enhancing Your Well-Being

As we age, the significance of a well-balanced and nutrient-rich diet becomes paramount. Nutrition plays a pivotal role in supporting overall health, managing chronic conditions, and ensuring vitality in the senior years. This chapter delves into the essential aspects of senior nutrition, offering practical guidance to help seniors make informed and wholesome choices for their well-being.

Understanding Changing Nutritional Needs

Caloric Requirements:

Metabolism tends to slow down with age, leading to a decrease in caloric requirements. However, the need for essential nutrients remains high. Seniors must focus on nutrient-dense foods to meet their nutritional needs without consuming excess calories.

Protein Intake:

Maintaining muscle mass is crucial for overall mobility and strength. Seniors should prioritize protein-rich foods such as lean meats, poultry, fish, eggs, and plant-based sources like legumes and tofu. Adequate protein intake supports muscle preservation and aids in the repair of tissues.

Calcium and Vitamin D:

Bone health becomes a focal point as individuals age. Calcium and vitamin D play pivotal roles in maintaining bone density. Dairy products, fortified plant-based milk, leafy greens, and exposure to sunlight are key sources of these essential nutrients.

Building a Balanced Plate

Colorful Fruits and Vegetables:

A rainbow of fruits and vegetables provides a spectrum of vitamins, minerals, and antioxidants. These nutrients contribute to immune health, skin integrity, and overall well-being. Aim for a variety of colors to ensure a diverse range of nutrients.

Whole Grains:

Choosing whole grains over refined grains provides fiber, which aids digestion and helps manage weight. Brown rice, quinoa, oats, and whole wheat products should be staples in a senior's diet.

Healthy Fats:

Incorporating sources of healthy fats, such as avocados, nuts, seeds, and olive oil, supports heart health and helps in the absorption of fat-soluble vitamins. Moderation is key, as fats are calorie-dense.

Managing Hydration

Dehydration Risks:

Seniors are often at a higher risk of dehydration due to various factors, including a reduced sensation of thirst. Staying hydrated is essential for maintaining cognitive function, supporting kidney health, and preventing constipation.

Hydrating Foods:

In addition to beverages, many fruits and vegetables have high water content and contribute to overall hydration. Water-rich foods like watermelon, cucumbers, and oranges can be enjoyable ways to stay hydrated.

Addressing Specific Nutrient Needs

Omega-3 Fatty Acids:

Omega-3 fatty acids, found in fatty fish like salmon, flaxseeds, and walnuts, support heart health and cognitive function. Including these foods in the diet can have long-term benefits for seniors.

Fiber for Digestive Health:

Adequate fiber intake aids in digestion, helps prevent constipation, and supports a healthy gut microbiome. Fiber-rich foods include whole grains, fruits, vegetables, and legumes.

Special Considerations for Chronic Conditions

Diabetes Management:

Seniors with diabetes must carefully manage their carbohydrate intake to regulate blood sugar levels. Working with a healthcare professional and a registered dietitian can help create a personalized plan.

Heart-Friendly Choices:

For those managing heart conditions, limiting sodium intake and choosing heart-healthy fats is crucial. Emphasizing a diet rich in fruits, vegetables, lean proteins, and whole grains supports cardiovascular health.

Meal Planning and Social Connection

Meal Preparation Tips:

Planning and preparing nutritious meals can be more challenging as we age. Simple strategies like batch cooking, using herbs and spices for flavor, and opting for nutrient-dense snacks can make mealtime more enjoyable and manageable.

Social Dining:

Eating is not only a physical necessity but also a social activity. Sharing meals with friends, family, or participating in community events fosters a sense of connection and joy. Social dining can enhance the overall dining experience and positively impact mental well-being.

The Role of Supplements

Vitamin and Mineral Supplements:

While it's ideal to obtain nutrients from whole foods, some seniors may benefit from supplements, especially if there are deficiencies or challenges in obtaining certain nutrients from food alone. Consulting with a healthcare professional before taking supplements is crucial to ensure safety and effectiveness.

Probiotics:

Probiotics, found in fermented foods like yogurt and kefir, contribute to gut health. Maintaining a healthy gut microbiome is increasingly recognized as vital for overall well-being and immune function.

Tailoring Nutrition to Individual Needs

Personalized Dietary Plans:

Each individual has unique nutritional needs based on factors like health conditions, medications, and lifestyle. Working with a registered dietitian can help seniors create personalized dietary plans that address their specific requirements and goals.

Mindful Eating:

Practicing mindful eating involves savoring each bite, paying attention to hunger and fullness cues, and being present during meals. This approach can enhance the dining experience and support overall digestive health.

Conclusion

Nutrition is a cornerstone of senior wellness, influencing physical health, mental well-being, and the overall quality of life. By understanding changing nutritional needs, building a balanced plate, and addressing specific nutrient requirements, seniors can proactively nurture their bodies and enhance their vitality beyond years. In the upcoming chapters, we will explore additional dimensions of senior wellness, including exercise routines, mental health strategies, and lifestyle choices that contribute to a fulfilling and active senior lifestyle. Remember, the journey to vitality is fueled by the choices we make each day, and a well-nourished body is better equipped to embrace the opportunities that lie ahead.

CHAPTER 4: STAYING ACTIVE AT EVERY AGE

Unlocking the Power of Movement for Senior Well-Being

Physical activity is the cornerstone of a vibrant and fulfilling senior life. As we age, staying active becomes increasingly important for maintaining mobility, supporting mental health, and preventing chronic conditions. This chapter explores the myriad benefits of exercise for seniors and provides practical guidance on incorporating enjoyable and effective physical activity into daily life.

Embracing the Benefits of Senior Exercise

Enhanced Mobility and Flexibility:

Regular exercise helps maintain joint flexibility and supports overall mobility. Engaging in activities that focus on stretching and range of motion can contribute to better flexibility, reducing the risk of injuries and enhancing daily functioning.

Improved Cardiovascular Health:

Cardiovascular exercises, such as walking, swimming, or cycling, contribute to heart health. These activities help maintain a healthy blood pressure, improve circulation, and enhance overall cardiovascular function.

Maintaining Healthy Weight:

Physical activity plays a crucial role in managing weight, especially as metabolism tends to slow down with age. Combining regular exercise with a balanced diet supports weight maintenance and overall well-being.

Muscle Strength and Bone Density:

Resistance training exercises, using weights or resistance bands, help preserve muscle mass and bone density. This is particularly vital for seniors to prevent falls, fractures, and maintain strength for daily activities.

Finding Joy in Movement

Tailoring Activities to Personal Preferences:

The key to sticking with an exercise routine is finding activities that bring joy. Whether it's dancing, gardening, swimming, or joining group fitness classes, seniors should explore and embrace activities that align with their interests and preferences.

Social Engagement through Exercise:

Exercise doesn't have to be a solitary endeavor. Joining group classes or walking clubs provides an opportunity for social interaction, reducing feelings of isolation and fostering a sense of community.

Incorporating Everyday Movement:

Everyday activities, such as walking the dog, gardening, or even household chores, contribute to overall physical activity. Finding ways to incorporate movement into daily routines is a practical and sustainable approach to staying active.

Designing a Balanced Exercise Routine

Cardiovascular Exercise:

Engaging in aerobic activities, such as brisk walking, swimming, or cycling, at least 150 minutes per week is recommended for seniors. This can be divided into shorter sessions throughout the week, making it more manageable.

Strength Training:

Incorporating strength training exercises at least two days a week is essential for preserving muscle mass. This can include using resistance bands, lifting weights, or practicing bodyweight exercises.

Flexibility and Balance Exercises:

Activities like yoga, tai chi, or specific balance exercises are beneficial for enhancing flexibility and stability. These exercises can reduce the risk of falls and improve overall body awareness.

Customizing for Health Conditions:

Seniors with specific health conditions, such as arthritis or heart disease, should tailor their exercise routine with guidance from healthcare professionals. Customized plans ensure safety and effectiveness in addressing individual needs.

Overcoming Barriers to Exercise

Addressing Joint Pain:

For those experiencing joint pain, low-impact activities like swimming or water aerobics can provide a gentler alternative. Seeking advice from healthcare professionals on pain management strategies is crucial for maintaining an active lifestyle.

Managing Chronic Conditions:

Seniors with chronic conditions, such as diabetes or osteoporosis, can benefit significantly from regular exercise. However, modifications may be necessary, and close collaboration with healthcare providers is essential to ensure safe and effective participation.

Nurturing Mental Well-Being Through Exercise

Cognitive Benefits:

Exercise has been linked to cognitive benefits, including improved memory and reduced risk of cognitive decline. Engaging in activities that challenge the mind, such as dancing or learning new exercises, enhances these cognitive benefits.

Mood Enhancement:

Physical activity triggers the release of endorphins, the "feel-good" hormones. Regular exercise is associated with a positive impact on mood, reducing symptoms of anxiety and depression in seniors.

Stress Reduction:

Exercise serves as a natural stress reliever. Whether it's a calming yoga session or a brisk walk in nature, physical activity helps reduce stress levels and promotes mental relaxation.

Incorporating Technology for Motivation

Fitness Apps and Wearables:

Technology can be a valuable ally in staying motivated. Fitness apps and wearables can help track activity levels, set goals, and provide a sense of accomplishment. Many of these tools are user-friendly and cater to various fitness levels.

Online Exercise Classes:

Virtual exercise classes offer the flexibility of working out from home. Many platforms provide a variety of classes, from gentle yoga to high-energy aerobics, catering to different preferences and fitness levels.

Safety Considerations and Precautions

Consulting Healthcare Professionals:

Before embarking on a new exercise routine, especially for those with pre-existing health conditions, consulting with healthcare professionals is paramount. They can offer guidance on safe activities and recommend any necessary precautions.

Listening to the Body:

Paying attention to the body's signals is crucial during exercise. Seniors should modify activities or seek guidance if they experience pain, dizziness, or any unusual symptoms during physical activity.

Conclusion

Staying active at every age is a powerful investment in senior well-being. Whether it's the joy of movement, the physical benefits of exercise, or the positive impact on mental health, regular physical activity is a key component of a vibrant and fulfilling senior life. In the upcoming chapters, we will explore additional dimensions of senior wellness, including strategies for mental health, preventive healthcare measures, and lifestyle choices that contribute to a holistic and active senior lifestyle. Remember, the journey to vitality is an ongoing process, and by embracing the power of movement, seniors can unlock a world of health, happiness, and longevity.

CHAPTER 5: MENTAL HEALTH AND COGNITIVE WELL-BEING

Nurturing the Mind for a Fulfilling Senior Life

As we age, the importance of mental health and cognitive well-being takes center stage. This chapter explores the intricacies of maintaining a healthy mind in the senior years, addressing the challenges and offering practical strategies to promote mental resilience, cognitive sharpness, and emotional well-being.

Recognizing the Importance of Mental Health

A Holistic View of Well-being:

Mental health is an integral component of overall well-being. It encompasses emotional, psychological, and social aspects, contributing to a person's ability to handle stress, form relationships, and make informed decisions. Nurturing mental health is vital for a fulfilling and vibrant senior life.

Addressing Mental Health Stigmas:

Unfortunately, societal stigmas around mental health can discourage open conversations. It's essential to challenge these stigmas and create an environment where seniors feel comfortable seeking support for their mental well-being.

The Aging Brain and Cognitive Function

Normal Aging vs. Cognitive Decline:

Normal aging involves subtle changes in cognitive function, such as a slight decline in processing speed and memory. However, distinguishing between normal aging and more serious cognitive decline, such as dementia or Alzheimer's disease, is crucial. Regular cognitive check-ups can aid in early detection and intervention.

Cognitive Reserve:

Engaging in mentally stimulating activities throughout life builds cognitive reserve, a concept suggesting that individuals with a higher cognitive reserve may better withstand age-related brain changes. Activities like reading, puzzles, and learning new skills contribute to cognitive reserve.

Strategies for Cognitive Well-being

Mental Stimulation:

Continuing to engage in mentally stimulating activities is vital for cognitive health. Reading, solving puzzles, playing musical instruments, or learning a new language are excellent ways to keep the mind active and agile.

Social Connection:

Maintaining social connections is not only beneficial for emotional well-being but also supports cognitive health. Regular social interactions, whether with family, friends, or community groups, provide opportunities for mental engagement and stimulation.

Lifelong Learning:

The pursuit of knowledge is a lifelong endeavor. Whether attending classes, joining discussion groups, or exploring online courses, seniors can continue learning and challenging their minds.

Managing Stress and Emotions

Stress Reduction Techniques:

Chronic stress can negatively impact both mental and physical health. Seniors should explore stress reduction techniques such as meditation, deep breathing exercises, or gentle yoga to promote relaxation and emotional well-being.

Emotional Expression:

Encouraging the expression of emotions is vital for mental health.

Whether through creative activities like writing or art, or through open communication with loved ones, expressing emotions helps maintain a healthy emotional balance.

Coping with Grief and Loss

Navigating Life Transitions:

Seniors often face significant life transitions, such as retirement, loss of a spouse, or changes in health. Acknowledging and navigating these transitions with support from friends, family, or professionals is crucial for emotional well-being.

Grief Support:

Seeking grief support, whether through counseling, support groups, or other resources, is essential for those experiencing loss. Grieving is a natural process, and having a supportive network can aid in coping with the emotions that accompany it.

The Role of Sleep in Mental Health

Quality Sleep Habits:

Adequate and restful sleep is foundational for mental health. Seniors should prioritize good sleep hygiene, including maintaining a consistent sleep schedule, creating a comfortable sleep environment, and addressing any sleep-related issues with healthcare professionals.

Addressing Sleep Disorders:

Conditions like insomnia or sleep apnea can significantly impact mental health. Seeking professional help to address and manage sleep disorders is essential for overall well-being.

Promoting Positive Self-esteem and Body Image

Embracing Aging:

Cultivating a positive self-image as one ages involves embracing the natural changes that come with time. Self-compassion and a focus on the wisdom and experience gained over the years contribute to a positive self-esteem.

Body Positivity:

Encouraging a positive body image involves recognizing and appreciating the body's capabilities rather than focusing on perceived flaws. Engaging in activities that promote physical well-being without unrealistic expectations contributes to a healthy body image.

Seeking Professional Support

Therapeutic Interventions:

Therapeutic interventions, such as counseling or psychotherapy, can provide valuable support for seniors facing mental health challenges. Trained professionals can offer guidance and strategies for coping with various emotional and psychological issues.

Medication Management:

For some individuals, medication may be a helpful component of mental health treatment. Consulting with healthcare professionals is essential to explore the potential benefits and risks associated with medication management.

Encouraging Active Lifestyle Choices

Balanced Nutrition:

Nutrition plays a crucial role in mental health. A balanced diet that includes essential nutrients, omega-3 fatty acids, and antioxidants supports cognitive function and emotional well-being.

Regular Physical Activity:

Exercise is not only beneficial for physical health but also has a profound impact on mental well-being. Regular physical activity releases endorphins, reduces stress, and enhances overall mood.

Conclusion

Nurturing mental health and cognitive well-being is a dynamic and ongoing process. By adopting strategies that stimulate the mind, managing stress, seeking support when needed, and making positive lifestyle choices, seniors can cultivate a resilient and thriving mental state. In the following chapters, we will explore additional dimensions of senior wellness, including preventive healthcare measures, social connections, and lifestyle choices that contribute to a holistic and active senior lifestyle. Remember, the journey to vitality involves both the body and the mind, and by prioritizing mental health, seniors can unlock the full spectrum of well-being in their later years.

CHAPTER 6: MANAGING CHRONIC CONDITIONS
Empowering Seniors for Optimal Health Despite Health Challenges

As individuals age, the likelihood of managing chronic health conditions increases. This chapter explores common chronic conditions affecting seniors, offers insights into effective management strategies, and provides guidance on maintaining overall well-being while living with chronic health challenges.

Understanding Common Chronic Conditions

Heart Disease:

Heart disease remains a prevalent concern among seniors. Conditions such as hypertension, coronary artery disease, and heart failure require ongoing management through lifestyle modifications, medication, and regular monitoring.

Diabetes:

Seniors may face challenges related to diabetes, a condition that impacts blood sugar levels. Managing diabetes involves a combination of dietary choices, medication adherence, and regular blood sugar monitoring.

Arthritis:

Arthritis, characterized by joint inflammation and stiffness, can affect mobility and quality of life. Seniors with arthritis benefit from a combination of gentle exercise, medication, and lifestyle adjustments to manage symptoms.

Osteoporosis:

Osteoporosis, characterized by weakened bones, increases the risk of fractures. Nutrition, weight-bearing exercises, and medications are key components of managing osteoporosis and preserving bone health.

Chronic Obstructive Pulmonary Disease (COPD):

COPD, which includes conditions like chronic bronchitis and emphysema, can impact respiratory function. Smoking cessation, medication management, and pulmonary rehabilitation are vital components of COPD management.

Lifestyle Strategies for Chronic Condition Management

Balanced Nutrition:

A well-balanced diet plays a crucial role in managing chronic conditions. For heart health, a diet low in saturated fats and sodium is recommended. Diabetics should focus on controlling carbohydrate intake, and arthritis sufferers may benefit from an anti-inflammatory diet rich in omega-3 fatty acids.

Regular Exercise:

Tailored exercise routines help manage various chronic conditions. Cardiovascular exercises, strength training, and flexibility exercises can be adapted to individual needs and capabilities. Consultation with healthcare professionals ensures safe and effective exercise plans.

Medication Adherence:

Adhering to prescribed medications is fundamental for managing chronic conditions. Seniors should communicate openly with healthcare providers about any challenges or concerns related to medications, such as side effects or financial constraints.

Regular Monitoring:

Frequent monitoring of key health indicators is crucial for managing chronic conditions. Regular blood pressure checks, glucose monitoring, bone density scans, and pulmonary function tests provide valuable insights into the effectiveness of management strategies.

Emotional Well-being and Chronic Illness

Coping Strategies:

Living with chronic conditions can be emotionally challenging. Developing coping strategies, such as mindfulness, relaxation techniques, or engaging in activities that bring joy, helps seniors navigate the emotional aspects of chronic illness.

Support Networks:

Building a strong support network is essential. Family, friends, and support groups provide emotional support and practical assistance. Sharing experiences with others facing similar challenges fosters a sense of understanding and camaraderie.

Mental Health Check-ins:

Regular check-ins with mental health professionals can be beneficial for seniors managing chronic conditions. Addressing any feelings of anxiety, depression, or emotional distress is integral to overall well-being.

Preventive Measures and Regular Check-ups

Vaccinations:

Seniors should stay up-to-date with vaccinations to prevent illness and complications. Influenza and pneumonia vaccinations, for example, are crucial for those with chronic conditions.

Routine Health Screenings:

Regular health screenings, tailored to individual health conditions, aid in early detection and prevention. Screenings may include cholesterol checks, eye exams, bone density tests, and cancer screenings.

Dental and Vision Care:

Good dental and vision care contribute to overall health. Regular dental check-ups and vision exams are important, as oral and visual health can impact nutrition, communication, and overall well-being.

Collaborating with Healthcare Professionals

Open Communication:

Effective communication with healthcare providers is key. Seniors should openly discuss symptoms, concerns, and any challenges faced in managing chronic conditions. This collaboration ensures personalized and effective care.

Care Coordination:

For seniors managing multiple chronic conditions, care coordination among healthcare providers is crucial. A cohesive approach ensures that all aspects of health are considered, and potential interactions between medications or treatments are addressed.

Lifestyle Adjustments for Specific Conditions

Heart-Healthy Lifestyle:

For those with heart conditions, lifestyle adjustments may include adopting a heart-healthy diet, engaging in regular cardiovascular exercise, and managing stress through relaxation techniques.

Diabetes Management:

Diabetics benefit from lifestyle adjustments that include monitoring carbohydrate intake, regular exercise, and medication management. Consistent blood sugar monitoring is crucial for effective diabetes management.

Arthritis-Friendly Lifestyle:

Seniors with arthritis may find relief through lifestyle adjustments such as gentle exercise, joint protection techniques, and assistive devices to support daily activities.

Osteoporosis Support:

Lifestyle adjustments for osteoporosis involve weight-bearing exercises, adequate calcium and vitamin D intake, and fall prevention strategies to reduce the risk of fractures.

COPD Management:

Seniors with COPD benefit from lifestyle adjustments that include smoking cessation, pulmonary rehabilitation, and strategies to conserve energy and manage shortness of breath.

Addressing Medication Challenges

Medication Management Strategies:

Managing medications can be complex, especially for seniors with multiple prescriptions. Strategies such as using pill organizers, setting reminders, and having regular medication reviews with healthcare providers ensure safe and effective medication management.

Over-the-Counter Medications:

Seniors should communicate with healthcare providers before taking over-the-counter medications, as they may interact with prescribed medications or exacerbate existing health conditions.

Engaging in Holistic Therapies

Complementary Therapies:

Complementary therapies, such as acupuncture, massage, or chiropractic care, may provide relief for some seniors managing chronic conditions. However, it's crucial to consult with healthcare providers before incorporating these therapies into a treatment plan.

Mind-Body Practices:

Mind-body practices, including meditation, yoga, or tai chi, can contribute to overall well-being. These practices offer physical and mental benefits, promoting relaxation and stress reduction.

Coping with End-of-Life Planning

Advance Directives:

Seniors should engage in conversations about end-of-life preferences and consider creating advance directives. This ensures that healthcare decisions align with personal values and wishes.

Hospice and Palliative Care:

Understanding and accessing hospice and palliative care options provides support for both seniors and their families during challenging times. These services focus on enhancing quality of life and comfort.

Conclusion

Managing chronic conditions is a dynamic and multifaceted process that requires collaboration, adaptation, and resilience. By embracing lifestyle adjustments, seeking support from healthcare professionals, and proactively managing both physical and emotional aspects of chronic illness, seniors can lead fulfilling lives despite health challenges. In the following chapters, we will explore additional dimensions of senior wellness, including social connections, preventive healthcare measures, and lifestyle choices that contribute to a holistic and active senior lifestyle. Remember, the journey to vitality is a comprehensive one, and by empowering themselves with knowledge and support, seniors can navigate the complexities of chronic conditions with grace and resilience.

CHAPTER 7: SOCIAL CONNECTIONS AND COMMUNITY ENGAGEMENT
Fostering Meaningful Relationships for a Rich and Fulfilling Senior Life

Social connections are a cornerstone of well-being, playing a pivotal role in the lives of seniors. This chapter explores the importance of social engagement, offers insights into building and maintaining meaningful relationships, and provides guidance on staying connected with the community for a vibrant and fulfilling senior life.

Recognizing the Impact of Social Connections on Health

Social Isolation and Health Risks:

Social isolation and loneliness can have profound effects on physical and mental health. Seniors experiencing social isolation may be at a higher risk of conditions such as cardiovascular disease, depression, and cognitive decline.

Positive Effects of Social Engagement:

Conversely, active social engagement is associated with numerous health benefits. Meaningful relationships can contribute to lower stress levels, improved immune function, and a sense of purpose and belonging.

Navigating Transitions and Building New Connections

Retirement and Lifestyle Adjustments:

The transition to retirement often involves lifestyle adjustments. Seniors should actively seek new social opportunities, such as joining clubs, taking classes, or participating in community events, to build a fulfilling post-retirement life.

Relocation and Community Integration:

For seniors who relocate, integrating into a new community

is essential for social well-being. Engaging with local groups, attending neighborhood events, and participating in community activities foster a sense of belonging.

Building and Maintaining Meaningful Relationships

Family Bonds:

Family relationships are a cornerstone of social support. Regular communication, spending quality time together, and celebrating milestones contribute to strong family bonds. Seniors can actively engage with family members, whether in person or through virtual means.

Friendships:

Nurturing friendships is vital for social well-being. Seniors should prioritize spending time with friends, whether through shared activities, regular phone calls, or virtual meet-ups. Meaningful friendships provide emotional support and companionship.

Romantic Relationships:

Maintaining romantic relationships in the senior years contributes to emotional fulfillment. Seniors can explore shared interests, engage in date nights, and foster open communication to strengthen romantic bonds.

Embracing Technology for Social Connection

Virtual Communication:

Technology offers valuable tools for staying connected. Video calls, social media, and messaging platforms enable seniors to connect with friends and family, regardless of geographical distances. Embracing technology broadens the scope of social engagement.

Online Communities:

Participating in online communities centered around shared interests provides an avenue for meeting new people and forming connections. Whether it's a book club, hobby group, or forum, online communities offer opportunities for social interaction.

Active Community Engagement

Local Clubs and Organizations:

Seniors can explore local clubs and organizations to connect with like-minded individuals. Whether it's a gardening club, a fitness class, or a volunteer group, these activities foster a sense of community and shared purpose.

Senior Centers:

Senior centers provide a hub for social activities, educational programs, and recreational events. Engaging with senior centers allows individuals to connect with peers, access resources, and participate in a variety of enriching activities.

Volunteer Opportunities:

Volunteering is a meaningful way to contribute to the community while forming connections. Seniors can explore volunteer opportunities aligned with their interests, skills, and time availability.

Intergenerational Programs:

Participating in intergenerational programs connects seniors with younger generations. Whether through mentoring, educational initiatives, or community projects, intergenerational interactions enrich the lives of all involved.

Nurturing Social Connections in Assisted Living or Care Facilities

Community Events:

Assisted living or care facilities often organize community events and activities. Seniors residing in such facilities can actively participate in these events, fostering a sense of community and camaraderie.

Group Activities:

Engaging in group activities, whether it's group exercise classes, arts and crafts sessions, or game nights, provides opportunities for social interaction within care facilities. These activities contribute to a supportive and vibrant living environment.

Family and Friend Visits:

Facilitating regular visits from family and friends is crucial for emotional well-being. Care facilities should encourage and support visits, whether in person or virtually, to maintain strong social connections for their residents.

Addressing Mobility and Transportation Challenges

Accessible Transportation:

Addressing transportation challenges is essential for maintaining social connections. Seniors should explore accessible transportation options within their community, such as senior transportation services or ride-sharing programs.

Community Support:

Communities can play a role in supporting seniors with mobility challenges. Initiatives such as volunteer-driven transportation services or community-sponsored events at easily accessible locations enhance social inclusion.

Fostering a Sense of Belonging

Community Inclusivity:

Communities should strive to be inclusive and welcoming to seniors. Creating age-friendly spaces, organizing events with a diverse range of activities, and fostering a sense of belonging contribute to the well-being of seniors.

Cultural and Spiritual Connections:

Seniors may find a sense of belonging through cultural or spiritual communities. Engaging in activities aligned with cultural or spiritual values provides a supportive network and shared experiences.

Coping with Grief and Loss

Grief Support Networks:

For seniors coping with grief and loss, having support networks is crucial. Joining grief support groups, engaging in counseling, and participating in memorial events provide avenues for expressing emotions and finding understanding.

Remembrance Rituals:

Creating personal rituals or participating in community remembrance events can be healing. These rituals provide opportunities to honor and remember loved ones while connecting with others who share similar experiences.

Encouraging Independence and Autonomy

Empowering Seniors:

Empowering seniors to maintain independence and autonomy in their social lives is essential. Encouraging them to make choices, participate in decision-making, and pursue activities they enjoy fosters a sense of control and well-being.

Respecting Individual Preferences:

Recognizing and respecting individual preferences for social engagement is vital. While some seniors may enjoy large social gatherings, others may prefer one-on-one interactions or smaller group settings. Tailoring social opportunities to individual preferences ensures a more meaningful experience.

Conclusion

Social connections are a cornerstone of a fulfilling and vibrant senior life. Whether through family bonds, friendships, community engagement, or online interactions, seniors can nurture meaningful relationships that contribute to their overall well-being. In the upcoming chapters, we will explore additional dimensions of senior wellness, including preventive healthcare measures, lifestyle choices, and strategies for maintaining a holistic and active senior lifestyle. Remember, the journey to vitality involves the heart, the mind, and the bonds we create with others, and by fostering social connections, seniors can embrace a life filled with companionship, joy, and shared experiences.

CHAPTER 8: PREVENTIVE HEALTHCARE MEASURES

Proactive Steps for Maintaining Senior Wellness

Preventive healthcare plays a pivotal role in promoting wellness and longevity in the senior years. This chapter explores the importance of proactive health measures, provides guidance on preventive screenings, vaccinations, and lifestyle choices, and empowers seniors to take charge of their health for a vibrant and thriving future.

Understanding the Significance of Preventive Healthcare

Proactive vs. Reactive Health Measures:

Preventive healthcare focuses on proactively identifying and addressing potential health issues before they become more serious. Seniors can benefit significantly from a preventive approach, which not only enhances quality of life but also reduces the burden of chronic conditions.

Health Screenings and Early Detection:

Regular health screenings are essential for early detection of potential health concerns. From cancer screenings to cardiovascular assessments, these screenings provide valuable insights into overall health and enable timely interventions.

Comprehensive Preventive Screenings for Seniors

Cardiovascular Screenings:

Cardiovascular health is paramount for seniors. Screenings such as blood pressure checks, cholesterol tests, and electrocardiograms (ECGs) help assess heart health and identify risk factors for cardiovascular diseases.

Cancer Screenings:

Routine cancer screenings, including mammograms, colonoscopies, and prostate exams, are crucial for early detection and treatment. These screenings play a key role in reducing the impact of various cancers on senior health.

Bone Density Tests:

Osteoporosis is a common concern for seniors, especially women. Bone density tests, such as dual-energy X-ray absorptiometry (DEXA) scans, assess bone health and help in the prevention of fractures.

Vision and Hearing Tests:

Regular vision and hearing tests are essential for maintaining sensory health. Detecting issues early allows for corrective measures, enhancing overall quality of life.

Diabetes Monitoring:

Seniors with diabetes should undergo regular monitoring of blood sugar levels. Hemoglobin A1c tests and regular glucose checks aid in managing diabetes and preventing complications.

Cognitive Assessments:

Cognitive screenings, such as memory tests and assessments for cognitive decline, are valuable for early detection of conditions like Alzheimer's disease. Early interventions and lifestyle adjustments can significantly impact cognitive health.

Vaccinations for Senior Wellness

Influenza (Flu) Vaccination:

Annual influenza vaccinations are recommended for seniors to protect against seasonal flu. The flu can have severe consequences for older individuals, and vaccination is a key preventive measure.

Pneumococcal Vaccination:

Pneumococcal vaccines help prevent pneumonia, a respiratory infection that can be particularly serious for seniors. Different types of pneumococcal vaccines are available, and seniors may need more than one dose.

Shingles Vaccination:

The shingles vaccine is recommended for seniors to prevent this painful condition caused by the varicella-zoster virus. Vaccination reduces the risk of developing shingles and postherpetic neuralgia.

Tetanus, Diphtheria, and Pertussis (Tdap) Vaccination:

Tdap vaccinations help protect against tetanus, diphtheria, and pertussis. Booster shots may be recommended, especially if it has been several years since the last vaccination.

COVID-19 Vaccination:

In the context of the ongoing COVID-19 pandemic, seniors should stay updated on COVID-19 vaccinations and follow recommendations from healthcare professionals and public health authorities.

Lifestyle Choices for Preventive Health

Balanced Nutrition:

A well-balanced diet is foundational for preventive health. Seniors should focus on nutrient-dense foods, including fruits, vegetables, lean proteins, and whole grains. Adequate hydration is also crucial for overall well-being.

Regular Physical Activity:

Engaging in regular exercise offers numerous health benefits. From maintaining a healthy weight to supporting cardiovascular health and reducing the risk of falls, physical activity is a cornerstone of preventive care.

Smoking Cessation:

Quitting smoking is one of the most impactful preventive measures for seniors. Smoking is linked to various health issues, including heart disease, respiratory conditions, and certain cancers.

Moderate Alcohol Consumption:

For those who consume alcohol, moderation is key. Excessive alcohol intake is associated with various health risks, including liver disease and an increased risk of accidents.

Stress Management:

Chronic stress can negatively impact both physical and mental health. Seniors should explore stress management techniques such as meditation, deep breathing exercises, and hobbies that promote relaxation.

Maintaining a Healthy Weight

Weight Management for Seniors:

Maintaining a healthy weight is crucial for preventing various health issues, including heart disease and diabetes. Seniors should focus on a balanced diet and regular exercise to manage and maintain their weight.

Body Mass Index (BMI) Awareness:

Understanding and monitoring body mass index (BMI) can help seniors assess whether they are in a healthy weight range. Healthcare professionals can provide guidance on achieving and maintaining a healthy BMI.

Routine Dental and Oral Health Care

Dental Check-ups:

Regular dental check-ups are essential for preventive oral care. Seniors should schedule routine visits to address issues like cavities, gum disease, and other oral health concerns.

Oral Hygiene Practices:

Maintaining good oral hygiene, including regular brushing and flossing, is vital for preventing dental issues. Proper oral care also contributes to overall health and well-being.

Eye Health and Regular Eye Exams

Routine Eye Exams:

Routine eye exams are crucial for maintaining vision health. Detecting issues such as cataracts, glaucoma, and macular degeneration early allows for appropriate interventions.

Corrective Measures:

For seniors with vision issues, corrective measures such as eyeglasses or contact lenses may be recommended. Following prescription guidelines and attending regular eye check-ups ensures optimal eye health.

Sleep Hygiene for Quality Rest

Establishing Healthy Sleep Habits:

Quality sleep is foundational for overall health. Seniors should prioritize establishing healthy sleep habits, including maintaining a consistent sleep schedule and creating a comfortable sleep environment.

Addressing Sleep Disorders:

Seniors experiencing sleep disorders, such as insomnia or sleep apnea, should seek professional help. Addressing sleep-related issues contributes to overall well-being.

Regular Health Check-ups and Assessments

Comprehensive Health Assessments:

Seniors should schedule regular health check-ups with healthcare providers. These assessments may include blood pressure checks, cholesterol tests, and discussions about overall health and well-being.

Medication Reviews:

Routine medication reviews with healthcare professionals ensure that prescriptions are current, effective, and aligned with overall health goals. Adjustments or changes may be made as needed.

Mental Health Check-ins and Support

Mental Health Awareness:

Seniors should prioritize mental health check-ins. Open communication with healthcare professionals about any feelings of anxiety, depression, or emotional distress ensures comprehensive well-being.

Counseling and Support Services:

Accessing counseling or support services can be beneficial for seniors facing mental health challenges. Trained professionals offer guidance and strategies for coping with various emotional and psychological issues.

Staying Informed and Empowered

Health Education:

Staying informed about current health guidelines, preventive measures, and lifestyle choices is empowering. Seniors should engage in health education programs, read reputable sources, and attend talks or seminars on relevant topics.

Advocating for Personal Health:

Seniors should actively advocate for their own health. This involves asking questions during healthcare visits, expressing concerns, and actively participating in decisions related to their well-being.

Conclusion

Preventive healthcare is the key to unlocking vitality and longevity in the senior years. By taking proactive steps, such as participating in screenings, getting vaccinated, making healthy lifestyle choices, and staying informed, seniors can empower themselves to lead fulfilling and vibrant lives. In the following chapters, we will continue to explore dimensions of senior wellness, including additional lifestyle choices, strategies for mental and emotional well-being, and a holistic approach to aging that embraces the full spectrum of health and happiness. Remember, the journey to vitality is an ongoing process, and by prioritizing preventive healthcare measures, seniors can navigate their later years with resilience, knowledge, and a commitment to their well-being.

CHAPTER 9: HOLISTIC APPROACHES TO AGING
Nurturing the Mind, Body, and Soul for a Balanced Senior Lifestyle

Aging is a multifaceted journey that encompasses not only physical health but also mental, emotional, and spiritual well-being. This chapter delves into holistic approaches to aging, exploring strategies for maintaining a balanced and fulfilling senior lifestyle that nourishes the mind, body, and soul.

The Holistic Framework for Senior Wellness

Mind-Body Connection:

Recognizing the interconnectedness of the mind and body is fundamental to holistic aging. Physical well-being influences mental health, and vice versa. By addressing both aspects, seniors can achieve a more balanced and comprehensive sense of wellness.

Embracing Emotional and Spiritual Dimensions:

Beyond physical and mental health, emotional and spiritual dimensions play crucial roles in the aging process. Cultivating a sense of purpose, finding joy in daily life, and connecting with one's inner self contribute to a holistic and meaningful senior lifestyle.

Mindful Aging and Self-Reflection

Mindful Practices:

Mindfulness involves being fully present in the moment, cultivating awareness without judgment. Seniors can embrace mindful practices, such as meditation, deep breathing exercises, and mindful walking, to foster a sense of calm and centeredness.

Self-Reflection:

Engaging in self-reflection allows seniors to explore their values, priorities, and goals. This introspective process provides insights into personal growth, fosters a sense of purpose, and encourages alignment with one's authentic self.

Creative Expression for Mental Well-being

Artistic Outlets:

Engaging in creative pursuits, such as painting, writing, or music, offers an outlet for self-expression and emotional release. Creative activities stimulate the mind, promote a sense of accomplishment, and contribute to overall mental well-being.

Journaling and Storytelling:

Keeping a journal or sharing personal stories provides an avenue for self-reflection and emotional expression. Seniors can document their experiences, memories, and reflections, creating a narrative that adds depth to their journey.

Cultivating a Positive Mindset

Positive Aging:

Shifting towards a positive mindset about aging is transformative. Embracing the wisdom and experiences gained over the years fosters a sense of gratitude and resilience. Seniors can focus on the positive aspects of aging, viewing it as a time of growth and self-discovery.

Gratitude Practices:

Practicing gratitude involves acknowledging and appreciating the positive aspects of life. Seniors can incorporate gratitude practices, such as keeping a gratitude journal or expressing thanks daily, to cultivate a positive outlook.

Spiritual Exploration and Connection

Spirituality in Aging:

Spirituality provides a framework for finding meaning and

purpose in life. Seniors may explore their spiritual beliefs, engage in practices that resonate with their values, and connect with a sense of the divine or transcendent.

Meditation and Contemplation:

Meditative practices, whether through prayer, mindfulness, or other contemplative techniques, offer seniors moments of inner stillness and connection. These practices contribute to a sense of peace and spiritual well-being.

Maintaining Social Connections

Interpersonal Relationships:

Social connections are integral to holistic well-being. Seniors should actively nurture relationships with family and friends, fostering a support network that contributes to emotional, mental, and even physical health.

Intergenerational Bonds:

Connecting with younger generations provides a sense of continuity and purpose. Whether through family gatherings, mentoring relationships, or community involvement, intergenerational bonds enrich the lives of seniors.

Nature and Outdoor Engagement

Nature as a Healing Force:

Spending time in nature has therapeutic benefits for seniors. Whether through walks in the park, gardening, or simply enjoying the outdoors, connecting with nature promotes relaxation, reduces stress, and enhances overall well-being.

Outdoor Activities:

Engaging in outdoor activities, such as gentle exercises, picnics, or birdwatching, allows seniors to stay active while enjoying the natural environment. Outdoor pursuits contribute to physical health and a sense of vitality.

Holistic Nutrition and Wellness

Nutrient-Rich Diets:

Holistic nutrition involves prioritizing whole, nutrient-dense foods that nourish the body. Seniors should focus on a well-balanced diet that includes a variety of fruits, vegetables, lean proteins, and whole grains to support overall health.

Mindful Eating Practices:

Mindful eating encourages a present awareness of the eating experience. Seniors can savor each bite, pay attention to hunger and fullness cues, and appreciate the flavors and textures of their meals for a more mindful approach to nutrition.

Holistic Fitness and Movement

Gentle Exercise Modalities:

Holistic fitness incorporates gentle exercise modalities that promote both physical and mental well-being. Practices such as yoga, tai chi, and qigong emphasize flexibility, balance, and mindful movement.

Balancing Strength and Flexibility:

Maintaining strength and flexibility is crucial for overall mobility and vitality. Seniors can engage in exercises that focus on building strength while also promoting flexibility, ensuring a holistic approach to physical well-being.

Holistic Approaches to Pain Management

Mind-Body Techniques:

Mind-body techniques, including meditation, guided imagery, and progressive muscle relaxation, can be effective in managing pain. These practices contribute to relaxation, reduce stress, and provide coping mechanisms for chronic pain.

Alternative Therapies:

Exploring alternative therapies, such as acupuncture, massage, or chiropractic care, offers seniors additional options for pain management. It's essential to consult with healthcare professionals to ensure the safety and appropriateness of these therapies.

Integrative Healthcare Practices

Combining Conventional and Complementary Approaches:

Integrative healthcare involves combining conventional medical approaches with complementary therapies. Seniors can work with healthcare providers to explore integrative options that align with their overall wellness goals.

Collaboration with Healthcare Professionals:

Effective communication with healthcare professionals is crucial in integrative healthcare. Seniors should openly discuss their preferences, experiences with complementary therapies, and explore collaborative approaches to well-being.

End-of-Life Planning and Legacy Building

Advance Care Planning:

Engaging in advance care planning allows seniors to express their preferences for end-of-life care. Discussions about medical decisions, hospice care, and funeral arrangements ensure that personal choices are respected.

Legacy Projects:

Seniors may consider engaging in legacy projects that reflect their values, experiences, and wisdom. This could include writing memoirs, creating family keepsakes, or contributing to community initiatives as a way of leaving a meaningful legacy.

Holistic Wellness Retreats and Programs

Wellness Retreats:

Participating in holistic wellness retreats provides seniors with immersive experiences that promote overall well-being. These retreats often include activities such as meditation, yoga, nutritional workshops, and opportunities for self-reflection.

Community Programs:

Community-based holistic wellness programs offer seniors accessible opportunities for engagement. These programs may include group activities, educational sessions, and support networks that contribute to a sense of community and well-being.

Conclusion

Holistic approaches to aging encompass the mind, body, and soul, recognizing the interconnected nature of these elements. By embracing mindful practices, nurturing social connections, exploring creative expressions, and tending to spiritual well-being, seniors can cultivate a balanced and fulfilling lifestyle that transcends the physical aspects of aging.

As we navigate the landscape of holistic aging, it's essential to recognize that every individual's journey is unique. What works for one person may differ for another, emphasizing the importance of personal exploration and customization. Seniors are encouraged to embrace a spirit of curiosity, openness, and self-discovery as they integrate holistic practices into their lives.

This chapter has illuminated various pathways to holistic well-being, encouraging seniors to view aging as a dynamic and evolving process. From the tranquility found in mindful practices to the vibrancy derived from creative expressions, each dimension contributes to the richness of the senior experience.

In the following chapters, we will delve further into the fabric of senior wellness, exploring additional lifestyle choices, strategies for mental and emotional well-being, and practical tips for adapting to the evolving landscape of aging. The journey towards vitality is an ongoing exploration, and by embracing holistic approaches, seniors can savor the depth and breadth of their later years with resilience, gratitude, and a profound connection to their inner selves.

CHAPTER 10: ADAPTING TO CHANGE AND EMBRACING RESILIENCE

Navigating Life Transitions and Flourishing in the Golden Years

Aging is a journey marked by transitions, both expected and unexpected. This chapter explores the art of adapting to change, fostering resilience, and embracing the opportunities for growth and fulfillment that each stage of life presents. Seniors can navigate transitions with grace, maintaining a positive outlook and savoring the richness of their golden years.

Acknowledging Life Transitions

Retirement as a New Beginning:

Retirement, while often anticipated, marks a significant transition. Seniors can approach this phase as a new beginning, embracing the freedom to explore personal interests, embark on new hobbies, and redefine their sense of purpose.

Health Challenges and Adaptation:

Adapting to changes in health is a common aspect of aging. Whether managing chronic conditions or facing unexpected health issues, seniors can cultivate resilience by actively participating in their care, seeking support, and maintaining a proactive approach to well-being.

Loss and Grief:

Navigating loss, whether the loss of a loved one, a role, or a cherished aspect of life, is a profound transition. Seniors can honor their grief, seek support through counseling or support groups, and explore ways to commemorate and celebrate the memories of what has been lost.

Cultivating Resilience

Positive Psychology and Resilience:

Positive psychology emphasizes the cultivation of strengths, positive emotions, and resilience. Seniors can integrate principles of positive psychology into their lives, focusing on gratitude, optimism, and adaptive coping strategies to navigate challenges.

Adapting to Change:

The ability to adapt to change is a cornerstone of resilience. Seniors can develop a flexible mindset, acknowledging that change is a natural part of life. By embracing adaptability, they empower themselves to navigate transitions with greater ease.

Staying Connected:

Maintaining social connections is a vital component of resilience. Seniors can draw on the support of friends, family, and community networks during times of change. Strengthening these connections fosters a sense of belonging and emotional well-being.

Finding Purpose and Meaning

Rediscovering Personal Passions:

Life transitions offer an opportunity to rediscover personal passions and interests. Seniors can explore hobbies, creative pursuits, or activities they've always wanted to try, infusing their lives with new sources of joy and purpose.

Contributing to Others:

Engaging in meaningful contributions to others fosters a sense of purpose. Whether through volunteering, mentoring, or sharing wisdom with younger generations, seniors can find fulfillment in making a positive impact on the lives of those around them.

Continued Learning and Growth:

The pursuit of knowledge and personal growth is a lifelong endeavor. Seniors can embrace continued learning through classes, workshops, or self-directed exploration, expanding their horizons and maintaining a vibrant intellectual life.

Embracing Technology for Connection

Digital Literacy and Connectivity:

Technology offers valuable tools for staying connected with the world. Seniors can embrace digital literacy, exploring social media, video calls, and online communities to maintain relationships, access information, and engage in virtual activities.

Online Learning Opportunities:

The internet provides a wealth of learning opportunities. Seniors can enroll in online courses, join virtual book clubs, or participate in webinars, accessing a world of knowledge from the comfort of their homes.

Telehealth and Healthcare Access:

Telehealth services have become increasingly accessible. Seniors can benefit from virtual healthcare appointments, consultations, and health monitoring, ensuring convenient and timely access to medical care.

Resilience in Care Facilities

Adjusting to Assisted Living or Nursing Homes:

Transitioning to assisted living or nursing homes can be a significant adjustment. Seniors and their families can work together to create a supportive environment, personalize living spaces, and maintain open communication with staff to ensure a positive experience.

Engaging in Facility Activities:

Participating in activities within care facilities contributes to a sense of community and purpose. Seniors can explore group activities, events, and outings organized by the facility, fostering social connections and enriching their daily lives.

Family and Friend Involvement:

Facilities should encourage family and friend involvement in the lives of their residents. Regular visits, both in-person and virtual, provide emotional support and maintain strong social connections, promoting the well-being of seniors in care.

Coping with Cognitive Changes

Maintaining Cognitive Health:

Cognitive changes are a natural part of aging, and seniors can take proactive steps to maintain cognitive health. Activities such as puzzles, brain games, and memory exercises contribute to mental stimulation and resilience.

Adaptive Strategies for Memory:

Seniors can employ adaptive strategies to manage changes in memory. This includes the use of memory aids, setting routines, and organizing living spaces to support cognitive function and promote independence.

Embracing Cognitive Support Services:

For seniors facing cognitive challenges, accessing support services is crucial. Memory care programs, cognitive therapy, and engaging in activities designed for cognitive well-being provide valuable assistance and enhance overall quality of life.

Coping with Loss and End-of-Life Transitions

Grief and Bereavement Support:

Coping with loss requires support and understanding. Seniors can benefit from grief counseling, bereavement groups, and other resources that offer solace and guidance during times of mourning.

End-of-Life Planning:

Open discussions about end-of-life preferences are essential. Seniors can engage in advanced care planning, clearly expressing their wishes regarding medical decisions, hospice care, and funeral arrangements. These conversations ensure that their choices are respected and followed.

Celebrating Life and Legacy:

In the face of life's transitions, seniors can celebrate their journey and leave a lasting legacy. Whether through creating memoirs, recording life stories, or participating in legacy projects, they can shape how they will be remembered and share the wisdom gained throughout their lives.

Adapting to Change with Dignity and Grace

Maintaining Dignity in Transitions:

Preserving dignity is paramount during life transitions. Seniors, families, and caregivers should approach changes with empathy, respect, and open communication. Providing choices and involving seniors in decision-making processes contributes to a sense of autonomy.

Accessible Resources for Transitions:

Access to resources and information eases the process of adapting to change. Seniors and their families can explore community services, support networks, and advocacy organizations that provide guidance and assistance throughout various transitions.

Holistic Well-Being in Later Years:

Adapting to change is an integral part of the holistic well-being of seniors. By approaching life transitions with resilience, purpose, and a commitment to growth, seniors can savor the richness of their later years, maintaining a positive outlook and embracing the opportunities each new phase brings.

Conclusion

Adapting to change is a lifelong skill, and as seniors navigate the intricacies of aging, they can do so with dignity, grace, and resilience. This chapter has explored the art of embracing life transitions, fostering resilience, and finding purpose and meaning in every stage. As we move forward, the subsequent chapters will delve into additional aspects of senior wellness, offering practical insights and guidance for a fulfilling and vibrant life. Remember, each transition is an opportunity for growth, and by approaching change with an open heart and a resilient spirit, seniors can continue to thrive in the golden years, embracing the beauty that comes with the passage of time.

CHAPTER 11: FOSTERING MENTAL AND EMOTIONAL WELL-BEING
Strategies for Cultivating Resilience, Joy, and Peace in Senior Life

Mental and emotional well-being is at the core of a fulfilling and vibrant senior life. This chapter explores various strategies to foster resilience, cultivate joy, and promote inner peace. From navigating the complexities of mental health to finding purpose and satisfaction in daily life, seniors can embrace practices that nurture their mental and emotional states.

Understanding Mental and Emotional Health in Seniors

The Importance of Mental Health:

Mental health is a vital component of overall well-being. Seniors should recognize the significance of mental health and actively engage in practices that support cognitive function, emotional balance, and psychological resilience.

Common Mental Health Challenges:

Seniors may encounter various mental health challenges, including depression, anxiety, and cognitive decline. Awareness of these challenges allows for early intervention and the implementation of strategies to maintain mental health.

Nurturing Resilience in the Face of Challenges

Cultivating Resilient Mindsets:

Resilience involves the ability to bounce back from adversity. Seniors can cultivate resilient mindsets by developing coping mechanisms, seeking support, and viewing challenges as opportunities for growth rather than insurmountable obstacles.

Mindfulness and Stress Reduction:

Mindfulness practices, such as meditation and deep breathing exercises, contribute to stress reduction. Seniors can integrate these techniques into their daily routines to promote emotional well-being and cultivate a sense of inner calm.

Adaptive Coping Strategies:

Adaptive coping involves the use of healthy strategies to navigate stressors. Seniors can develop personalized coping mechanisms, such as maintaining social connections, engaging in hobbies, or seeking professional support when needed.

Finding Joy and Purpose in Daily Life

Discovering Meaningful Activities:

Seniors can find joy by engaging in activities that bring fulfillment and satisfaction. Whether it's pursuing hobbies, volunteering, or spending time with loved ones, discovering meaningful pursuits adds purpose to daily life.

Creative Expressions for Joy:

Creative activities, such as art, music, or writing, provide an outlet for self-expression and joy. Seniors can explore their creative sides, fostering a sense of accomplishment and delight in the process.

Celebrating Milestones and Achievements:

Acknowledging personal milestones and achievements is essential. Seniors should take time to celebrate their accomplishments, both big and small, fostering a positive outlook and a sense of pride in their life journey.

Building and Maintaining Social Connections

The Impact of Social Connections on Mental Health:

Social connections play a crucial role in mental health. Seniors should prioritize building and maintaining relationships, as social interactions contribute to a sense of belonging, reduce feelings of isolation, and provide emotional support.

Family Bonds and Support Systems:

Family relationships serve as a foundational support system. Seniors can strengthen family bonds through regular communication, shared activities, and the exchange of emotional support, contributing to a positive and connected family dynamic.

Friendships and Companionship:

Nurturing friendships is equally important. Seniors should invest time and effort into building and sustaining meaningful friendships, enjoying companionship and shared experiences with those who bring joy to their lives.

Holistic Approaches to Mental Health

Nutrition and Brain Health:

Nutrition plays a role in cognitive function. Seniors can adopt a brain-healthy diet, including foods rich in antioxidants, omega-3 fatty acids, and vitamins that support cognitive health.

Physical Exercise and Cognitive Function:

Regular physical exercise has cognitive benefits. Seniors can engage in activities that promote cardiovascular health, strength, and flexibility, contributing to improved cognitive function and mental well-being.

Quality Sleep for Mental Wellness:

Adequate and quality sleep is essential for mental wellness. Seniors should prioritize establishing healthy sleep habits, ensuring restful sleep that supports cognitive function and emotional balance.

Addressing Mental Health Challenges

Recognizing Signs of Depression:

Seniors and their caregivers should be aware of signs of depression, including persistent sadness, loss of interest in activities, and changes in sleep patterns. Seeking professional help is crucial if depression is suspected.

Anxiety Management Strategies:

Anxiety can manifest in various forms. Seniors can explore anxiety management strategies, such as relaxation techniques, cognitive-behavioral therapy, and support groups, to address and cope with anxious feelings.

Cognitive Decline and Memory Care:

For seniors experiencing cognitive decline, memory care programs and cognitive therapies provide specialized support. Early interventions and engaging activities tailored to cognitive abilities contribute to a higher quality of life.

Integrating Technology for Mental Stimulation

Digital Brain Games and Apps:

Technology offers opportunities for mental stimulation. Seniors can explore digital brain games and apps designed to challenge cognitive abilities, enhancing memory, attention, and problem-solving skills.

Online Learning Platforms:

Virtual learning platforms provide access to a wide range of courses and educational resources. Seniors can engage in online learning to stimulate their minds, explore new subjects, and stay intellectually active.

Social Media and Virtual Connections:

Social media platforms facilitate virtual connections. Seniors can use these tools to stay in touch with friends and family, join online communities, and participate in discussions that contribute to mental stimulation.

Seeking Professional Support

Therapeutic Interventions:

Therapeutic interventions, such as counseling and psychotherapy, offer valuable support for mental health. Seniors can benefit from professional guidance to navigate life challenges, manage emotions, and build resilience.

Psychiatric Care and Medication Management:

In cases where psychiatric care is necessary, seniors should work with healthcare professionals to explore medication management options. A comprehensive approach that considers both therapy and medication can address mental health challenges effectively.

Support Groups and Community Resources:

Support groups provide a sense of community and understanding. Seniors can explore local and online support groups, connecting with others facing similar challenges and sharing experiences that contribute to emotional well-being.

Holistic Approaches to Emotional Well-being

Mind-Body Practices for Emotional Balance:

Mind-body practices, such as yoga, tai chi, and qigong, contribute to emotional balance. Seniors can incorporate these gentle exercises into their routines, promoting relaxation and a harmonious mind-body connection.

Expressive Arts Therapies:

Expressive arts therapies, including art therapy and music therapy, offer outlets for emotional expression. Seniors can engage in these therapeutic modalities to process emotions, enhance self-awareness, and foster emotional well-being.

Nature and Emotional Restoration:

Spending time in nature has emotional benefits. Seniors can enjoy outdoor activities, walks in nature, or gardening, harnessing the restorative power of natural environments for emotional well-being.

Building Emotional Resilience

Embracing Change and Acceptance:

Emotional resilience involves embracing change and cultivating acceptance. Seniors can work on adapting to new circumstances, letting go of unrealistic expectations, and finding contentment in the present moment.

Emotional Intelligence:

Developing emotional intelligence allows seniors to navigate relationships and emotions effectively. Seniors can engage in practices that enhance self-awareness, empathy, and effective communication, contributing to positive emotional connections.

Mindfulness and Emotional Regulation:

Mindfulness practices extend to emotional regulation. Seniors can use mindfulness techniques to observe and manage their emotional responses, fostering a balanced and mindful approach to their inner states.

Cultivating Inner Peace and Serenity

Mindful Meditation Practices:

Mindful meditation practices promote inner peace. Seniors can explore meditation techniques that focus on breath awareness, guided imagery, or body scan meditations, creating moments of tranquility and mental clarity.

Spiritual Exploration for Peace:

Spiritual exploration contributes to a sense of peace and purpose. Seniors can engage in practices aligned with their spiritual beliefs, whether through prayer, meditation, or participation in spiritual communities.

Gratitude and Contentment:

Cultivating gratitude enhances inner peace. Seniors can incorporate gratitude practices into their daily lives, reflecting on the positive aspects of each day and fostering contentment with the present.

Integrating Holistic Approaches

Holistic Lifestyle Choices:

Integrating holistic lifestyle choices contributes to overall mental and emotional well-being. Seniors can adopt a holistic approach by combining healthy nutrition, regular exercise, mindfulness practices, and social engagement.

Personalized Well-being Plans:

Creating personalized well-being plans allows seniors to tailor strategies to their unique needs. Working with healthcare professionals, seniors can develop plans that address mental health, emotional well-being, and overall life satisfaction.

Life Review and Reflection:

Engaging in life review and reflection is a therapeutic process. Seniors can explore their life stories, acknowledge achievements and challenges, and gain insights that contribute to a sense of closure and fulfillment.

Conclusion

Fostering mental and emotional well-being is a continual journey, and this chapter has provided a comprehensive guide for seniors to navigate this path with resilience, joy, and peace. By understanding the intricacies of mental health, adopting adaptive coping strategies, and embracing practices that nurture emotional balance, seniors can savor the richness of their inner lives in the golden years.

In the following chapters, we will continue to explore dimensions of senior wellness, including physical health, lifestyle choices, and practical tips for a thriving and vibrant life. Remember, prioritizing mental and emotional well-being is a gift to oneself, contributing to a fulfilling and meaningful senior experience.

CHAPTER 12: EMBRACING A VIBRANT AND ACTIVE LIFESTYLE

Strategies for Physical Fitness, Leisure, and Social Engagement

Maintaining a vibrant and active lifestyle is the key to unlocking the full potential of senior years. This chapter explores strategies for physical fitness, leisure activities, and social engagement that contribute to overall vitality and well-being. From tailored exercise routines to fulfilling leisure pursuits, seniors can embrace an active lifestyle that enriches their golden years.

The Importance of Physical Activity for Seniors

Physical Activity and Aging:

Physical activity is fundamental to healthy aging. Seniors should recognize the benefits of staying physically active, including improved cardiovascular health, enhanced flexibility, and increased energy levels.

The Role of Exercise in Well-being:

Regular exercise plays a crucial role in overall well-being. Seniors can experience physical, mental, and emotional benefits, including reduced risk of chronic diseases, improved mood, and enhanced cognitive function.

Tailoring Exercise Routines for Seniors

Consultation with Healthcare Professionals:

Before starting a new exercise routine, seniors should consult with healthcare professionals. A thorough health assessment ensures that the chosen exercises align with individual health needs and any existing medical conditions.

Aerobic Exercises for Cardiovascular Health:

Aerobic exercises, such as brisk walking, swimming, or cycling, contribute to cardiovascular health. Seniors can incorporate these activities into their routines to improve heart health, endurance, and overall fitness.

Strength Training for Muscle Health:

Strength training exercises build and maintain muscle mass. Seniors can include resistance training, weightlifting, or bodyweight exercises to enhance strength, support joint health, and improve overall mobility.

Flexibility and Balance Exercises:

Flexibility and balance exercises are essential for preventing falls and maintaining mobility. Seniors can practice activities like yoga or tai chi to enhance flexibility, balance, and coordination.

Low-Impact Exercises for Joint Health:

Low-impact exercises, such as swimming or elliptical training, provide cardiovascular benefits with reduced impact on joints. Seniors can choose activities that are gentle on the joints, promoting long-term joint health.

Incorporating Exercise into Daily Life

Active Daily Routines:

Simple lifestyle changes can increase daily physical activity. Seniors can choose stairs over elevators, engage in household chores, and take short walks, integrating movement into their daily routines.

Walking and Nature Exploration:

Walking is an accessible and enjoyable form of exercise. Seniors can explore nearby parks, nature trails, or neighborhoods, enjoying the health benefits of walking while connecting with the outdoors.

Group Exercise Classes:

Group exercise classes provide a social and supportive environment. Seniors can join classes tailored to their fitness level, such as water aerobics, senior fitness classes, or dance classes, fostering camaraderie and motivation.

Leisure Activities for Mental and Emotional Well-being

Engaging Hobbies and Interests:

Leisure activities contribute to mental and emotional well-being. Seniors can pursue hobbies and interests, such as reading, gardening, or crafting, providing a source of joy, relaxation, and creative expression.

Cultural and Artistic Pursuits:

Exploring cultural and artistic pursuits adds richness to life. Seniors can attend concerts, visit museums, or participate in art classes, immersing themselves in cultural experiences that stimulate the mind and foster creativity.

Travel and Exploration:

Traveling and exploring new places offer exciting opportunities. Seniors can embark on local or international adventures, discovering new cultures, cuisines, and landscapes, fostering a sense of curiosity and adventure.

Social Engagement and Community Involvement

Community Centers and Senior Programs:

Community centers and senior programs provide a hub for social engagement. Seniors can participate in group activities, events, and workshops, connecting with peers and expanding their social circles.

Volunteering and Community Service:

Volunteering offers a sense of purpose and community contribution. Seniors can explore volunteer opportunities aligned with their interests, making a positive impact and enjoying the social connections that come with community service.

Joining Social Clubs and Groups:

Social clubs and groups cater to various interests. Seniors can join book clubs, gardening groups, or game nights, fostering friendships and staying socially connected through shared activities.

Technology and Virtual Socialization

Online Social Platforms:

Technology facilitates virtual socialization. Seniors can use online platforms for video calls, social media, and virtual events, staying connected with friends and family, especially when in-person interactions may be limited.

Virtual Classes and Webinars:

Virtual classes and webinars offer learning opportunities and social interaction. Seniors can enroll in online courses, attend virtual workshops, and participate in discussions, expanding their knowledge while connecting with others.

Gaming and Cognitive Engagement:

Gaming platforms provide cognitive engagement and social interaction. Seniors can explore games that challenge the mind, participate in online multiplayer games, and connect with a broader gaming community.

Active Aging Communities and Living Environments

Active Aging Communities:

Active aging communities offer tailored environments for seniors. These communities often provide amenities such as fitness centers, walking trails, and group activities, creating a supportive and active living environment.

Senior-Friendly Infrastructure:

Creating a senior-friendly living environment is essential. Seniors can choose housing with features like accessible walkways, well-lit spaces, and community areas, promoting safe and active living.

Accessible Fitness Facilities:

Accessible fitness facilities cater to the unique needs of seniors. Seniors can choose gyms or wellness centers equipped with senior-friendly exercise machines, adaptive equipment, and knowledgeable staff.

Embracing Intergenerational Connections

Family Involvement:

Involvement with family members fosters intergenerational connections. Seniors can participate in family gatherings, share stories and experiences, and engage with younger generations, creating a sense of continuity and mutual understanding.

Mentoring and Sharing Wisdom:

Seniors have valuable life experiences to share. Mentoring relationships provide an opportunity for seniors to share their wisdom with younger individuals, creating meaningful connections and contributing to the broader community.

Intergenerational Programs:

Intergenerational programs bring different age groups together. Seniors can participate in programs that involve collaboration with schools, community organizations, or youth groups, fostering connections and bridging generational gaps.

Maintaining Independence and Adaptability

Accessible Transportation Options:

Maintaining independence often involves accessible transportation. Seniors can explore transportation options that cater to their needs, ensuring they can engage in activities and remain connected to their communities.

Adapting Activities to Abilities:

Adapting activities to individual abilities is crucial. Seniors should choose exercises and leisure pursuits that align with their physical capabilities, ensuring a positive and sustainable approach to an active lifestyle.

Home Modifications for Safety:

Home modifications contribute to safety and independence.

Seniors can assess their living spaces, making adjustments such as installing handrails, improving lighting, and creating accessible layouts to support independent living.

Conclusion

Embracing a vibrant and active lifestyle is a transformative choice that empowers seniors to live their golden years with vitality and joy. From tailored exercise routines to engaging leisure activities and social connections, every aspect contributes to the holistic well-being of seniors.

In the subsequent chapters, we will explore practical tips for everyday living, share insights on nutritional choices, and provide guidance on navigating healthcare decisions. The journey to vitality continues, and by embracing an active lifestyle, seniors can savor the richness of each moment, ensuring a fulfilling and purposeful senior experience.

CHAPTER 13: PRACTICAL TIPS FOR EVERYDAY LIVING

Navigating Daily Challenges with Ease and Confidence

Practical tips for everyday living are invaluable for seniors as they navigate the various facets of daily life. This chapter provides insights and strategies to enhance convenience, safety, and overall well-being in daily activities. From home organization to time management, seniors can adopt practical approaches that contribute to a smooth and enjoyable lifestyle.

Creating an Accessible and Comfortable Living Space

Home Safety Assessments:

Conducting a home safety assessment is a proactive measure. Seniors can identify potential hazards, such as loose rugs or uneven flooring, and make necessary adjustments to create a safer living environment.

Decluttering and Organizing:

Decluttering living spaces reduces the risk of falls and enhances accessibility. Seniors can organize their homes, removing unnecessary items, and creating clear pathways to move comfortably and safely.

Accessible Furniture and Layouts:

Choosing accessible furniture and layouts promotes ease of movement. Seniors can opt for chairs with proper support, adjustable beds, and layouts that minimize the need for excessive bending or reaching.

Time Management and Organization

Daily Routines and Schedules:

Establishing daily routines and schedules provides structure. Seniors can create a daily plan that includes dedicated times for meals, activities, and rest, fostering a sense of predictability and routine.

Utilizing Calendars and Reminders:

Calendars and reminders assist in staying organized. Seniors can use physical calendars, digital apps, or smart devices to set reminders for appointments, medication schedules, and other important events.

Prioritizing Tasks:

Prioritizing tasks helps manage time effectively. Seniors can identify essential tasks and prioritize them, ensuring that important responsibilities are addressed while minimizing stress.

Nutritional Choices for Optimal Health

Balanced and Nutrient-Rich Diets:

Maintaining a balanced and nutrient-rich diet is crucial. Seniors should include a variety of fruits, vegetables, lean proteins, and whole grains in their meals, supporting overall health and well-being.

Hydration Practices:

Staying hydrated is essential for health. Seniors can establish hydration routines, keeping water accessible throughout the day and incorporating hydrating foods, such as fruits and soups, into their diet.

Meal Planning and Preparation:

Meal planning and preparation streamline nutrition. Seniors can plan meals in advance, ensuring a variety of nutrients, and consider batch cooking or utilizing meal delivery services for added convenience.

Mobility and Independence

Assistive Devices and Mobility Aids:

Assistive devices enhance mobility and independence. Seniors can explore options like canes, walkers, or mobility scooters based on their individual needs, improving confidence in daily movements.

Accessible Clothing and Footwear:

Choosing accessible clothing and footwear simplifies dressing. Seniors can opt for clothing with easy closures, elastic waistbands, and comfortable shoes that provide stability and support.

Fall Prevention Strategies:

Implementing fall prevention strategies is paramount. Seniors can use non-slip mats, install grab bars in bathrooms, and wear proper footwear to reduce the risk of falls and enhance overall safety.

Cognitive Well-being and Memory Support

Memory Aids and Techniques:

Memory aids and techniques assist in daily tasks. Seniors can use tools like reminder notes, calendars, and smartphone apps to support memory and stay organized.

Creating Memory-Friendly Environments:

Creating memory-friendly environments minimizes confusion. Seniors can use labels, color-coded systems, and visual cues to make their living spaces more navigable and supportive of cognitive well-being.

Engaging in Mental Stimulation:

Engaging in mental stimulation activities is essential. Seniors can participate in puzzles, brain games, reading, and social interactions to keep their minds active and sharp.

Social Connection and Emotional Well-being

Regular Communication with Loved Ones:

Regular communication with loved ones is vital. Seniors can stay connected through phone calls, video chats, or in-person visits, nurturing relationships and combating feelings of isolation.

Participating in Social Activities:

Participating in social activities fosters a sense of community. Seniors can join clubs, attend social events, or volunteer, enjoying the companionship and emotional support that social engagement provides.

Embracing Emotional Resilience:

Embracing emotional resilience is crucial for well-being. Seniors can develop coping mechanisms, seek support when needed, and engage in activities that bring joy and fulfillment, contributing to emotional well-being.

Healthcare Management and Advocacy

Regular Health Check-ups:

Regular health check-ups are essential for preventive care. Seniors should schedule routine medical appointments, screenings, and vaccinations to monitor and maintain their health.

Medication Management Strategies:

Medication management is crucial for seniors on multiple prescriptions. Seniors can use pill organizers, set alarms, or enlist the help of caregivers to ensure they take medications as prescribed.

Open Communication with Healthcare Providers:

Open communication with healthcare providers is key. Seniors should actively engage in discussions about their health, ask questions, and express any concerns, fostering a collaborative approach to healthcare.

Financial Management and Security

Budgeting and Financial Planning:

Budgeting and financial planning contribute to stability. Seniors can create budgets, track expenses, and consider consulting with financial advisors to ensure a secure financial future.

Protecting Against Financial Scams:

Protecting against financial scams is essential. Seniors should be cautious about sharing personal information, verify the legitimacy of requests, and seek guidance from trusted sources to prevent scams.

Legal and Estate Planning:

Legal and estate planning provide peace of mind. Seniors can create wills, establish power of attorney, and make decisions about their estates, ensuring that their wishes are documented and respected.

Technology Adoption for Convenience

Smart Home Devices for Accessibility:

Smart home devices enhance accessibility. Seniors can explore options like voice-activated assistants, smart thermostats, and home security systems to make their living spaces more convenient and user-friendly.

Telehealth Services:

Telehealth services offer convenient healthcare options. Seniors can explore virtual consultations, remote monitoring, and telemedicine appointments, ensuring access to healthcare from the comfort of their homes.

Online Shopping and Services:

Online shopping and services simplify daily tasks. Seniors can use online platforms for grocery shopping, medication refills, and various services, saving time and effort in their daily lives.

Transportation Options for Independence

Accessible Transportation Services:

Accessible transportation services support independence. Seniors can explore options such as senior transportation programs, ride-sharing services, or community transportation to ensure they can move around conveniently.

Driving Safety and Assessments:

Driving safety is crucial for those who still drive. Seniors should undergo regular driving assessments, stay informed about traffic rules, and consider alternative transportation when needed.

Community Involvement and Transportation:

Community involvement often requires transportation. Seniors can coordinate with local community centers, senior programs, or volunteer services to access transportation options for social activities and events.

Conclusion

Navigating daily life with confidence and ease is a key aspect of senior well-being. This chapter has provided practical tips and strategies for seniors to enhance their everyday living experience, promoting safety

CHAPTER 14: NAVIGATING HEALTHCARE DECISIONS AND ADVOCACY

Empowering Seniors to Make Informed Health Choices

As seniors navigate the complex landscape of healthcare, informed decision-making and advocacy become essential components of maintaining well-being. This chapter provides insights and strategies to empower seniors in making healthcare decisions, navigating medical systems, and advocating for their health needs. From understanding healthcare options to fostering effective communication with healthcare providers, seniors can take an active role in their health journey.

Understanding Healthcare Options

Medicare and Medicaid:

Understanding Medicare and Medicaid is crucial for seniors. Seniors should be familiar with the coverage, eligibility criteria, and enrollment processes for these government-sponsored healthcare programs.

Private Insurance Plans:

Seniors may opt for private insurance plans. It's essential to explore various insurance options, comparing coverage, premiums, and out-of-pocket costs to find a plan that aligns with individual health needs.

Supplemental Insurance:

Supplemental insurance can enhance coverage. Seniors may consider supplemental plans to address gaps in their primary insurance, providing additional benefits for specific healthcare services.

Building a Healthcare Support Team

Primary Care Physicians:

Establishing a relationship with a primary care physician is foundational. Seniors should choose a healthcare provider they trust, who understands their medical history, and who can coordinate overall healthcare needs.

Specialists and Allied Health Professionals:

Consulting specialists and allied health professionals is essential for specialized care. Seniors may need the expertise of specialists such as cardiologists, endocrinologists, or physical therapists to address specific health concerns.

Care Coordinators and Case Managers:

Care coordinators or case managers assist in navigating healthcare systems. Seniors can work with these professionals to coordinate appointments, manage medications, and ensure seamless communication between healthcare providers.

Effective Communication with Healthcare Providers

Preparing for Medical Appointments:

Preparation is key for medical appointments. Seniors should compile a list of questions, bring relevant medical records, and communicate any changes in symptoms or concerns to make the most of their appointments.

Open and Honest Communication:

Open and honest communication fosters understanding. Seniors should feel comfortable discussing their health concerns, sharing relevant information about their lifestyle, and asking questions to clarify any uncertainties.

Advocating for Personal Health Goals:

Advocating for personal health goals ensures personalized care. Seniors can communicate their preferences, values, and health priorities to healthcare providers, contributing to a collaborative approach in decision-making.

Managing Medications Effectively

Understanding Prescriptions:

Understanding prescriptions is crucial for medication management. Seniors should be aware of the purpose, dosage, and potential side effects of their medications, seeking clarification from healthcare providers when needed.

Creating Medication Lists:

Maintaining a comprehensive medication list aids in organization. Seniors can create a detailed list that includes medication names, dosages, and schedules, facilitating accurate communication with healthcare providers.

Medication Reviews and Adjustments:

Regular medication reviews are important. Seniors should participate in medication reviews with healthcare providers, discussing any changes in their health status or potential side effects to ensure appropriate adjustments.

Preventive Care and Screenings

Importance of Preventive Care:

Prioritizing preventive care contributes to overall health. Seniors should schedule regular check-ups, screenings, and vaccinations, addressing potential health issues before they escalate.

Cancer Screenings and Detection:

Cancer screenings are crucial for early detection. Seniors should follow recommended cancer screening guidelines, including mammograms, colonoscopies, and prostate screenings, based on individual risk factors.

Immunizations for Seniors:

Immunizations protect against preventable diseases. Seniors should stay up-to-date with vaccinations, including flu shots, pneumonia vaccines, and other immunizations recommended for their age group.

Chronic Disease Management

Understanding Chronic Conditions:

Understanding chronic conditions is essential for management. Seniors with chronic diseases such as diabetes, hypertension, or arthritis should work closely with healthcare providers to develop effective management plans.

Lifestyle Modifications for Chronic Health:

Lifestyle modifications play a key role. Seniors can adopt healthy habits, such as regular exercise, balanced nutrition, and stress management, to complement medical interventions for chronic conditions.

Support Groups and Peer Networks:

Support groups provide emotional support. Seniors with chronic conditions can join support groups or peer networks, sharing experiences, coping strategies, and insights with others facing similar health challenges.

Advanced Care Planning

Advance Directives and Living Wills:

Advance directives outline healthcare preferences. Seniors should create advance directives and living wills, clearly stating their preferences for medical interventions, end-of-life care, and decision-makers in case they cannot communicate their wishes.

Healthcare Power of Attorney:

Designating a healthcare power of attorney is crucial. Seniors should appoint a trusted individual to make healthcare decisions on their behalf if they become incapacitated, ensuring their wishes are respected.

Discussions with Family and Healthcare Providers:

Open discussions with family and healthcare providers are necessary. Seniors should communicate their advanced care plans with their loved ones and healthcare team, fostering a shared understanding of their preferences.

Accessing Home Healthcare and Rehabilitation Services

Home Healthcare Options:

Home healthcare services support recovery. Seniors can explore options such as home nursing, physical therapy, or occupational therapy when recovering from illnesses or surgeries, allowing them to receive care in the comfort of their homes.

Rehabilitation and Physical Therapy:

Rehabilitation and physical therapy aid in recovery. Seniors undergoing surgeries or managing chronic conditions can benefit from rehabilitation services, improving mobility, strength, and overall functional independence.

Assistive Devices and Adaptive Equipment:

Assistive devices enhance independence at home. Seniors can explore adaptive equipment such as grab bars, shower chairs, or mobility aids to create a safe and supportive living environment.

Long-Term Care Planning

Understanding Long-Term Care Options:

Understanding long-term care options is crucial for future planning. Seniors should explore options such as assisted living, nursing homes, or in-home care, considering their preferences, financial resources, and potential long-term care needs.

Long-Term Care Insurance:

Long-term care insurance provides financial support. Seniors may consider long-term care insurance as a way to cover potential costs associated with extended healthcare needs, ensuring financial stability for future care.

Legal and Financial Planning for Long-Term Care:

Legal and financial planning is integral to long-term care. Seniors should engage in discussions with legal and financial advisors to create plans that align with their long-term care preferences and financial situation.

End-of-Life Care Considerations

Hospice and Palliative Care:

Hospice and palliative care focus on comfort and quality of life. Seniors facing serious illnesses may benefit from hospice or palliative care services, providing support for both physical and emotional well-being.

Family Discussions on End-of-Life Preferences:

Open discussions with family about end-of-life preferences are essential. Seniors should communicate their wishes regarding end-of-life care, burial or cremation preferences, and any religious or cultural considerations with their loved ones.

Legal Documentation for End-of-Life Decisions:

Legal documentation ensures end-of-life wishes are honored. Seniors should work with legal professionals to create documents such as a durable power of attorney for healthcare, ensuring that their chosen decision-maker can advocate for their preferences.

Conclusion

Navigating healthcare decisions and advocacy empowers seniors to take control of their health journey. This chapter has provided comprehensive insights and strategies for seniors to make informed decisions, communicate effectively with healthcare providers, and plan for various aspects of their health and well-being.

In the subsequent chapters, we will explore additional dimensions of senior wellness, including social engagement, lifestyle choices, and practical tips for a fulfilling senior experience. By embracing a proactive approach to healthcare decisions, seniors can enhance their quality of life and cultivate a sense of empowerment in their golden years.

CHAPTER 15: CULTIVATING SOCIAL CONNECTIONS AND COMMUNITY ENGAGEMENT

Nurturing Relationships and Active Participation in Later Life

Social connections and community engagement play a pivotal role in the well-being of seniors. This chapter explores the importance of cultivating relationships, participating in social activities, and contributing to the community. From fostering connections with family and friends to engaging in local initiatives, seniors can experience the enriching benefits of a socially active and vibrant lifestyle.

Recognizing the Importance of Social Connections

Impact on Mental and Emotional Well-being:

Social connections have a profound impact on mental and emotional well-being. Seniors who maintain strong social ties often experience lower rates of depression, increased resilience, and improved overall life satisfaction.

Physical Health Benefits:

Social engagement contributes to physical health. Seniors who are socially active may experience lower blood pressure, reduced risk of chronic diseases, and enhanced immune system function, promoting longevity and vitality.

Cognitive Stimulation:

Social interactions provide cognitive stimulation. Engaging in conversations, participating in group activities, and sharing experiences with others contribute to cognitive health, potentially reducing the risk of cognitive decline.

Nurturing Family Relationships

Quality Time with Loved Ones:

Quality time with family is invaluable. Seniors can prioritize spending time with children, grandchildren, and extended family members, fostering strong bonds and creating lasting memories.

Interactions Across Generations:

Interactions across generations are enriching. Seniors can share their experiences, wisdom, and stories with younger family members, creating a sense of continuity and connection between different age groups.

Family Traditions and Celebrations:

Family traditions and celebrations strengthen ties. Seniors can actively participate in family rituals, celebrations, and holidays, contributing to a sense of belonging and familial connection.

Fostering Friendships and Social Circles

Maintaining Existing Friendships:

Maintaining existing friendships is important. Seniors can stay in touch with longtime friends through phone calls, letters, or social media, ensuring that these meaningful connections endure over time.

Making New Friends:

Making new friends contributes to social diversity. Seniors can explore social clubs, hobby groups, or community events to meet like-minded individuals and form new connections in their communities.

Socializing through Shared Interests:

Socializing through shared interests enhances connections. Seniors can join clubs, classes, or groups that align with their hobbies and passions, fostering friendships with those who share similar interests.

Engaging in Community Activities

Community Volunteering:

Community volunteering provides a sense of purpose. Seniors can contribute their time and skills to local charities, schools, or organizations, making a positive impact on their communities and experiencing the fulfillment of giving back.

Participation in Local Events:

Participating in local events fosters community ties. Seniors can attend fairs, festivals, and community gatherings, enjoying the camaraderie of shared experiences and celebrating the vibrancy of their neighborhoods.

Involvement in Civic Groups:

Involvement in civic groups promotes active citizenship. Seniors can join civic organizations, neighborhood associations, or community councils, actively participating in discussions and initiatives that shape their local communities.

Utilizing Technology for Social Connection

Online Social Platforms:

Technology facilitates virtual socialization. Seniors can use online platforms for video calls, social media, and virtual events, staying connected with friends and family members, especially when in-person interactions may be limited.

Virtual Classes and Workshops:

Virtual classes and workshops offer learning opportunities. Seniors can enroll in online courses, attend virtual workshops, and participate in discussions, expanding their knowledge while connecting with others in the digital space.

Online Gaming Communities:

Online gaming communities provide social interaction. Seniors can explore online games that cater to their interests, connecting with a broader gaming community and enjoying the social aspects of multiplayer games.

Participating in Senior Centers and Programs

Senior Centers as Social Hubs:

Senior centers serve as social hubs. Seniors can explore local senior centers that offer a variety of activities, classes, and events, providing opportunities to socialize with peers and engage in recreational pursuits.

Educational and Recreational Programs:

Participating in educational and recreational programs is enriching. Seniors can attend workshops, lectures, and classes at senior centers, fostering continuous learning and connecting with others who share similar interests.

Fitness and Wellness Classes:

Fitness and wellness classes contribute to holistic well-being. Seniors can join exercise classes, yoga sessions, or wellness programs at senior centers, promoting physical health while socializing with fellow participants.

Supporting and Engaging with Others

Mentorship Opportunities:

Mentorship opportunities create meaningful connections. Seniors can offer mentorship to younger individuals, sharing their knowledge and experiences, while also benefiting from the sense of fulfillment that comes with guiding others.

Peer Support Groups:

Peer support groups provide understanding and empathy. Seniors facing similar challenges, whether health-related or life transitions, can join peer support groups, offering and receiving support within a compassionate community.

Active Listening and Emotional Support:

Active listening fosters emotional connections. Seniors can practice active listening in their interactions, offering emotional support to friends and peers, creating an environment where individuals feel heard and understood.

Organizing and Hosting Social Gatherings

Hosting Social Events:

Hosting social events strengthens community ties. Seniors can organize gatherings, potlucks, or themed events, creating opportunities for neighbors and friends to come together and enjoy each other's company.

Celebrating Milestones and Achievements:

Celebrating milestones enhances social bonds. Seniors can commemorate birthdays, anniversaries, or personal achievements with friends and family, creating occasions for joy and shared happiness.

Cultural and Hobby-based Gatherings:

Cultural and hobby-based gatherings foster connections. Seniors can organize events centered around shared interests, such as book clubs, art exhibitions, or music nights, creating spaces for cultural enrichment and socialization.

Overcoming Social Barriers and Isolation

Transportation Solutions:

Transportation solutions enhance accessibility. Seniors facing transportation challenges can explore community transportation options, volunteer-driven services, or coordinate carpools to overcome barriers and participate in social activities.

Addressing Mobility Limitations:

Addressing mobility limitations is essential. Seniors with mobility challenges can seek accessible venues, utilize mobility aids, or explore virtual events to ensure they can actively engage in social activities.

Community Outreach and Inclusivity:

Community outreach promotes inclusivity. Seniors can advocate for community initiatives that address social isolation, working with local organizations to create inclusive environments and support networks.

Conclusion

Cultivating social connections and community engagement is an integral aspect of a fulfilling senior experience. This chapter has explored various strategies for seniors to nurture relationships, participate in community life, and overcome potential barriers to socialization.

In the following chapters, we will continue to explore dimensions of senior wellness, including lifestyle choices, practical tips, and overall strategies for a vibrant and purposeful life. By actively embracing social connections, seniors can contribute to the vitality of their communities and savor the richness of their later years.

CHAPTER 16: NOURISHING BODY AND MIND: HOLISTIC APPROACHES TO SENIOR NUTRITION

Balancing Nutritional Needs for Optimal Well-being

Nutrition plays a pivotal role in the health and vitality of seniors. This chapter explores the importance of senior nutrition, focusing on balanced dietary choices, hydration, and mindful eating practices. From understanding nutritional requirements to practical tips for meal planning, seniors can embrace holistic approaches to nourish both body and mind in their golden years.

The Significance of Senior Nutrition

Impact on Physical Health:

Senior nutrition has a direct impact on physical health. A well-balanced diet supports essential bodily functions, contributes to optimal organ function, and aids in the prevention of chronic diseases commonly associated with aging.

Influence on Cognitive Function:

Nutrition influences cognitive function. Seniors who prioritize a nutrient-rich diet may experience improved memory, sharper cognitive skills, and a reduced risk of cognitive decline, promoting mental acuity in later life.

Role in Emotional Well-being:

Nutrition plays a role in emotional well-being. A healthy diet can positively impact mood, reduce the risk of depression, and contribute to an overall sense of emotional resilience, enhancing the quality of life for seniors.

Understanding Senior Nutritional Needs

Essential Nutrients for Seniors:

Seniors require a mix of essential nutrients to support their health. These include vitamins such as B12 and D, minerals like calcium and potassium, protein, fiber, and healthy fats, each playing a specific role in maintaining well-being.

Caloric Requirements and Metabolism:

Caloric requirements may change with age. Seniors should be mindful of their metabolism, adjusting their caloric intake to account for changes in activity levels, muscle mass, and overall energy expenditure.

Hydration Needs:

Proper hydration is vital. Seniors may be at an increased risk of dehydration, making it essential to maintain adequate fluid intake, which can come from water, herbal teas, soups, and hydrating fruits and vegetables.

Building a Balanced Plate for Senior Wellness

Incorporating Fruits and Vegetables:

Fruits and vegetables are nutritional powerhouses. Seniors should aim to fill half their plate with colorful fruits and vegetables, as they provide essential vitamins, minerals, antioxidants, and fiber for digestive health.

Choosing Whole Grains:

Whole grains offer sustained energy. Seniors can opt for whole grains like brown rice, quinoa, and whole wheat, which provide fiber, vitamins, and minerals while contributing to heart health and maintaining steady blood sugar levels.

Prioritizing Lean Proteins:

Lean proteins are crucial for muscle health. Seniors can include sources like poultry, fish, beans, and tofu, which provide essential amino acids and support muscle maintenance and repair.

Incorporating Healthy Fats:

Healthy fats support overall health. Seniors can choose sources like avocados, nuts, olive oil, and fatty fish, which contribute to heart health, brain function, and the absorption of fat-soluble vitamins.

Monitoring Sodium Intake:

Sodium moderation is essential. Seniors should be mindful of their salt intake to manage blood pressure, opting for fresh herbs, spices, and other flavorings to enhance the taste of meals without relying on excessive salt.

Practical Tips for Senior Meal Planning

Regular, Balanced Meals:

Regular, balanced meals provide stability. Seniors should aim for three well-balanced meals each day, incorporating a mix of nutrients to meet their daily nutritional needs.

Snacking with Purpose:

Purposeful snacking supports energy levels. Seniors can choose nutrient-dense snacks, such as yogurt with berries, whole-grain crackers with cheese, or fresh fruit, to maintain energy levels between meals.

Mindful Eating Practices:

Mindful eating enhances the dining experience. Seniors can practice mindful eating by savoring each bite, paying attention to hunger and fullness cues, and appreciating the flavors and textures of their meals.

Variety in Food Choices:

Variety ensures a range of nutrients. Seniors should include a diverse selection of foods in their diet, trying different fruits, vegetables, proteins, and grains to maximize nutritional intake.

Adapting to Dietary Preferences and Restrictions:

Adapting meals to preferences and restrictions is key. Seniors can tailor their diets to accommodate dietary preferences, allergies, or medical restrictions, ensuring that their nutritional needs are met while enjoying the foods they love.

Special Considerations for Senior Nutrition

Calcium and Vitamin D for Bone Health:

Calcium and vitamin D are critical for bone health. Seniors should incorporate dairy products, fortified plant-based milk, leafy greens, and sunlight exposure to support bone density and reduce the risk of fractures.

B12 Supplementation for Vegetarians:

Vegetarian seniors may need B12 supplementation. As B12 is primarily found in animal products, vegetarians should consider B12 supplements or fortified foods to prevent deficiencies that can affect energy levels and neurological function.

Fiber for Digestive Health:

Adequate fiber promotes digestive health. Seniors can include fiber-rich foods like whole grains, fruits, vegetables, and legumes in their diet to prevent constipation and support a healthy digestive system.

Reducing Added Sugars:

Limiting added sugars is essential. Seniors can minimize the consumption of sugary beverages, sweets, and processed foods, choosing natural sources of sweetness like fruits to maintain overall health and reduce the risk of chronic diseases.

Managing Chronic Conditions through Nutrition:

Nutrition plays a role in managing chronic conditions. Seniors with conditions such as diabetes, hypertension, or heart disease can work with healthcare providers and dietitians to create personalized nutrition plans that support their health goals.

Hydration Practices for Senior Wellness

Importance of Hydration:

Proper hydration is vital for health. Seniors should recognize the importance of staying hydrated to support bodily functions, maintain cognitive function, and prevent complications related to dehydration.

Hydration Monitoring:

Monitoring hydration levels is crucial. Seniors can pay attention to signs of dehydration, such as dark urine, dry mouth, or dizziness, and adjust their fluid intake accordingly, especially in hot weather or during physical activity.

Hydrating Foods and Beverages:

Hydrating foods complement fluid intake. Seniors can include water-rich foods like melons, cucumbers, and soups in their meals, and choose hydrating beverages such as water, herbal teas, and diluted fruit juices.

Strategies for Overcoming Nutritional Challenges

Appetite Changes and Small, Frequent Meals:

Appetite changes are common. Seniors experiencing reduced appetite can opt for smaller, more frequent meals throughout the day to ensure they meet their nutritional needs.

Dental Health Considerations:

Dental health impacts food choices. Seniors with dental challenges can choose soft, easy-to-chew foods, and explore options like smoothies, soups, and nutrient-rich shakes to ensure they receive essential nutrients.

Addressing Digestive Issues:

Digestive issues may require adjustments. Seniors experiencing digestive discomfort can work with healthcare professionals to identify trigger foods, explore dietary modifications, and ensure they receive adequate nutrition.

Seeking Guidance from Healthcare Professionals:

Professional guidance is invaluable. Seniors should consult with healthcare professionals, including registered dietitians, to receive personalized nutrition advice based on their health status, dietary preferences, and any existing medical conditions.

Integrating Culinary Enjoyment into Senior Living

Cooking for Pleasure and Socialization:

Cooking can be a joyful activity. Seniors can engage in cooking for pleasure, experimenting with new recipes, and involving friends or family members, turning meal preparation into a social and enjoyable experience.

Exploring Culinary Workshops and Classes:

Culinary workshops offer learning opportunities. Seniors can participate in cooking classes or workshops that cater to their interests, expanding their culinary skills and knowledge while connecting with others who share a passion for food.

Gardening for Fresh, Homegrown Ingredients:

Gardening promotes a connection to food. Seniors with access to outdoor space can explore gardening, cultivating fresh herbs, vegetables, or fruits, and incorporating homegrown ingredients into their meals for added freshness and flavor.

Conclusion

Nourishing the body and mind through holistic nutrition is a cornerstone of senior well-being. This chapter has delved into the significance of senior nutrition, providing practical tips, dietary considerations, and strategies to overcome challenges, ensuring that seniors can embrace a balanced and fulfilling approach to their dietary choices.

In the upcoming chapters, we will continue to explore various facets of senior wellness, including lifestyle choices, practical tips for everyday living, and strategies for maintaining vitality beyond the years. By fostering a mindful approach to nutrition, seniors can savor the pleasures of culinary enjoyment while supporting their overall health and vitality.

Certainly! Here's an in-depth Chapter 17 for your ebook, "Vitality Beyond Years: A Comprehensive Guide to Health and Wellness for Seniors."

CHAPTER 17: EMBRACING FULFILLMENT AND JOY IN YOUR SENIOR YEARS

Crafting a Purposeful and Joyful Life Beyond Retirement

As we conclude this guide to health and wellness for seniors, the focus shifts to embracing fulfillment and joy in the golden years. This chapter explores the importance of finding purpose, maintaining a positive mindset, and pursuing activities that bring joy and satisfaction. By cultivating a sense of purpose and joy, seniors can navigate retirement with enthusiasm, making the most of their experiences and contributing to a fulfilling senior life.

The Power of Purpose in Senior Living

Defining Personal Meaning and Goals:

Finding purpose involves defining personal meaning and goals. Seniors can reflect on their values, passions, and aspirations, identifying activities and pursuits that bring a sense of fulfillment and contribute to their overall well-being.

Engaging in Meaningful Activities:

Meaningful activities foster purpose. Seniors can engage in volunteer work, mentorship, or community involvement, contributing their skills and experiences to make a positive impact, creating a sense of purpose beyond personal fulfillment.

Cultivating Lifelong Learning:

Lifelong learning contributes to purpose. Seniors can embrace opportunities for continuous education, whether through formal courses, workshops, or self-directed learning, expanding their knowledge and skills, and maintaining a curious and engaged mindset.

Nurturing Emotional Well-being

Mindfulness and Gratitude Practices:

Mindfulness enhances emotional well-being. Seniors can incorporate mindfulness practices and gratitude exercises into their daily routines, promoting a positive outlook, reducing stress, and fostering appreciation for the present moment.

Building and Maintaining Social Connections:

Social connections contribute to emotional health. Seniors can prioritize relationships with family, friends, and community members, creating a supportive network that provides companionship, understanding, and emotional support.

Coping Strategies for Life Transitions:

Life transitions may require coping strategies. Seniors facing changes in health, living arrangements, or relationships can benefit from coping mechanisms such as seeking support, practicing resilience, and adapting to new circumstances with a positive mindset.

Pursuing Joyful Activities and Hobbies

Rediscovering and Exploring Hobbies:

Rediscovering hobbies brings joy. Seniors can revisit past hobbies or explore new interests, whether it's painting, gardening, playing music, or engaging in creative pursuits, creating avenues for self-expression and enjoyment.

Cultural and Recreational Enjoyment:

Cultural and recreational activities enrich life. Seniors can attend concerts, visit museums, participate in community events, or explore outdoor activities, immersing themselves in experiences that bring joy, cultural enrichment, and a sense of adventure.

Travel and Exploration in Retirement:

Traveling enhances retirement experiences. Seniors can embrace the opportunity to explore new destinations, whether locally or internationally, experiencing different cultures, cuisines, and landscapes, and creating lasting memories.

Maintaining Physical Vitality

Staying Active with Enjoyable Exercises:

Enjoyable exercises support physical vitality. Seniors can choose exercises that bring joy, such as dancing, swimming, or nature walks, making physical activity a pleasurable part of their routine while promoting cardiovascular health and flexibility.

Yoga and Mindful Movement Practices:

Yoga and mindful movement contribute to well-being. Seniors can explore gentle yoga, tai chi, or other mindful movement practices that enhance flexibility, balance, and mental focus, promoting physical and mental vitality.

Holistic Approaches to Health:

Holistic health practices offer a comprehensive approach. Seniors can explore complementary therapies such as acupuncture, massage, or aromatherapy, incorporating these practices into their wellness routine to address both physical and emotional well-being.

Crafting a Fulfilling Lifestyle

Balancing Independence and Support:

Balancing independence and support is key. Seniors can assess their needs and preferences, making informed decisions about living arrangements, support services, and community involvement to create a lifestyle that aligns with their values.

Culinary Enjoyment and Healthy Eating:

Culinary enjoyment contributes to a fulfilling lifestyle. Seniors can savor the pleasures of cooking, dining, and exploring diverse cuisines, creating a connection to food that enhances overall well-being while prioritizing nutritional choices.

Financial Wellness and Retirement Planning:

Financial wellness ensures peace of mind. Seniors can engage in prudent financial planning, considering budgeting, investments, and retirement plans to secure their financial future, providing a foundation for a fulfilling and worry-free lifestyle.

Embracing Technology for Connection and Learning

Connecting with Loved Ones Through Technology:

Technology fosters connection. Seniors can utilize smartphones, tablets, and video calls to stay connected with family and friends, bridging geographical distances and maintaining meaningful relationships through virtual communication.

Online Learning Opportunities:

Online learning offers accessible education. Seniors can explore virtual courses, webinars, and educational platforms to continue learning and expanding their knowledge, embracing the convenience of online resources for personal growth.

Exploring Virtual Entertainment:

Virtual entertainment enhances leisure activities. Seniors can enjoy movies, concerts, or cultural events through online platforms, accessing a variety of entertainment options from the comfort of their homes, broadening their cultural experiences.

Reflecting on Life's Journey and Legacy

Legacy Reflection and Documentation:

Reflecting on life's journey is a meaningful practice. Seniors can engage in legacy reflection, documenting their experiences, values, and life lessons for future generations, creating a tangible legacy that preserves their unique story.

Sharing Wisdom and Experiences:

Sharing wisdom contributes to a sense of purpose. Seniors can mentor younger generations, participate in storytelling initiatives, or engage in intergenerational activities, passing down knowledge and experiences that contribute to a sense of legacy.

Celebrating Personal Milestones:

Celebrating milestones enhances joy. Seniors can commemorate birthdays, anniversaries, and personal achievements, taking the time to reflect on their journey, express gratitude, and surround themselves with the love and appreciation of friends and family.

Navigating End-of-Life Considerations with Grace

Advance Care Planning and End-of-Life Wishes:

Advance care planning ensures personal preferences are honored. Seniors can engage in discussions about end-of-life wishes, create advance directives, and designate healthcare proxies, providing clarity for themselves and their loved ones.

Embracing Palliative and Hospice Care:

Palliative and hospice care focus on comfort. Seniors facing serious illnesses can explore palliative and hospice care options, receiving compassionate support that prioritizes physical, emotional, and spiritual well-being during the final stages of life.

Creating Meaningful End-of-Life Moments:

Creating meaningful moments is a final gift. Seniors can participate in activities that bring joy and fulfillment in their final days, surrounded by loved ones and creating cherished memories that celebrate a life well-lived.

Conclusion: Embracing the Fullness of Senior Life

In concluding this guide, we celebrate the rich tapestry of senior life—a journey marked by resilience, wisdom, and the continual pursuit of well-being. The chapters have explored health, social connections, nutrition, purpose, and joy, providing a holistic roadmap for seniors to navigate their later years with vitality.

As you embrace the fullness of your senior life, may you find purpose, joy, and fulfillment

CHAPTER 18: EMBRACING THE FULLNESS OF SENIOR LIFE - A RECAP

In this concluding chapter, we reflect on the comprehensive journey through "Vitality Beyond Years: A Comprehensive Guide to Health and Wellness for Seniors." The guide has served as a roadmap, offering insights, strategies, and practical tips to empower seniors in cultivating a holistic approach to their well-being.

The Essence of Senior Wellness Explored

1. **Health and Wellness Foundations:** We began by laying the foundations of senior wellness, emphasizing the importance of regular health check-ups, preventive care, and the proactive management of chronic conditions. The goal was to empower seniors to take charge of their physical health.

2. **Mental and Emotional Well-being:** Addressing mental and emotional well-being was a key theme. Seniors were encouraged to foster resilience, engage in activities that promote cognitive health, and seek support when facing life transitions or emotional challenges.

3. **Social Connections and Community Engagement:** Recognizing the significance of social connections, we explored strategies for seniors to nurture relationships with family and friends, engage in community activities, and leverage technology for virtual connections, fostering a vibrant social life.

4. **Nutrition and Hydration Practices:** The guide delved into the intricacies of senior nutrition, emphasizing the role of balanced meals, hydration, and mindful eating in promoting physical and cognitive health. Special considerations and practical tips were provided to

address unique nutritional needs.

5. **Cultivating Joy and Purpose:** Understanding the power of joy and purpose, seniors were encouraged to explore activities that bring fulfillment, whether through hobbies, cultural experiences, travel, or engaging in lifelong learning. The chapter highlighted the importance of maintaining a positive mindset and emotional well-being.

6. **Technology and Modern Living:** Seniors were guided on harnessing the benefits of technology for connection, learning, and entertainment. The chapter underscored the role of virtual platforms in maintaining relationships, accessing educational resources, and enjoying cultural experiences from the comfort of home.

7. **Legacy Reflection and End-of-Life Considerations:** The guide explored the reflective practice of legacy building, providing insights into sharing wisdom, celebrating milestones, and navigating end-of-life considerations with grace. Seniors were encouraged to engage in advance care planning to ensure their preferences are honored.

Embracing the Fullness of Senior Life

The concluding chapter encourages seniors to embrace the fullness of their lives, celebrating the richness of experiences, relationships, and the wisdom gained over the years. It emphasizes the importance of finding joy, purpose, and fulfillment in every moment.

As seniors navigate their later years, the guide encourages them to reflect on their unique journey, prioritize well-being, and savor the pleasures of life. Whether through social connections, meaningful activities, or embracing the technological advancements of the modern age, seniors are empowered to live with vitality beyond their years.

In the spirit of embracing the fullness of senior life, this guide stands as a companion—a source of information, inspiration, and practical guidance. May seniors find continued health, joy, and fulfillment as they navigate the beautiful tapestry of their senior years.

www.ingramcontent.com/pod-product-compliance
Lightning Source LLC
Chambersburg PA
CBHW060748260726

48660CB00002B/524